How to Sleep Better

CRAFTED BY SKRIUWER

Copyright © 2024 by Skriuwer.
All rights reserved. No part of this book may be used or reproduced in any form whatsoever without written permission except in the case of brief quotations in critical articles or reviews.

For more information, contact : **kontakt@skriuwer.com** (www.skriuwer.com)

TABLE OF CONTENTS

CHAPTER 1: THE BASICS OF SLEEP

- Understanding why rest is vital for the body and mind
- Short-term and long-term effects of not sleeping well
- Simple first steps to improve nightly rest

CHAPTER 2: UNDERSTANDING SLEEP STAGES

- Overview of Non-REM and REM patterns
- Deep sleep vs. light sleep differences
- Tips to support each stage for better rest

CHAPTER 3: COMMON SLEEP PROBLEMS

- Identifying insomnia, apnea, restless legs, and more
- Signs that may indicate you need more help
- Basic strategies to address frequent issues

CHAPTER 4: THE LINK BETWEEN SLEEP AND STRESS

- How stress chemicals affect rest
- Recognizing worry loops that keep you awake
- Stress-reducing methods to calm the mind before bed

CHAPTER 5: BUILDING A GOOD SLEEP ENVIRONMENT

- Setting the right temperature and lighting
- Reducing noise and clutter
- Choosing supportive mattresses and bedding

CHAPTER 6: IMPACT OF TECHNOLOGY ON SLEEP

- How blue light and mental stimulation affect rest
- Managing device use before bed
- Finding a healthy balance with modern gadgets

CHAPTER 7: NUTRITION AND SLEEP

- How diet influences rest quality
- Timing of meals and smart snack choices
- Caffeine and alcohol guidelines

CHAPTER 8: IMPORTANCE OF EXERCISE

- How physical activity supports better rest
- Choosing the right time and intensity for workouts
- Simple daily movement ideas

CHAPTER 9: EFFECTS OF LIGHT

- Natural vs. artificial light on circadian rhythms
- Reducing evening brightness for smoother bedtime
- Seasonal changes and helpful light strategies

CHAPTER 10: THE ROLE OF ROUTINE

- Why stable schedules help the body's clock
- Building morning, afternoon, and bedtime habits
- Handling weekends and social events

CHAPTER 11: SLEEP MYTHS

- Common misconceptions that harm rest
- Sorting fact from fiction about snoring and nap ideas
- Adjusting beliefs to support healthier nights

CHAPTER 12: SLEEP AND MOOD

- The close link between emotions and rest
- How sadness, worry, and anger disrupt sleep
- Ways to protect mood and get better nights

CHAPTER 13: SLEEPING POSITIONS

- Pros and cons of back, side, and stomach postures
- Using pillows to support alignment
- Special cases, such as expecting or back pain

CHAPTER 14: NAPPING

- Different nap lengths and their effects
- Timing naps to avoid harming nighttime rest
- Handling naps for shift workers or busy days

CHAPTER 15: CHANGING YOUR THINKING ABOUT SLEEP

- Replacing negative beliefs with balanced ones
- Overcoming performance pressure at bedtime
- Simple mental exercises for a calmer mind

CHAPTER 16: SLEEP ACROSS DIFFERENT AGES

- Infants, children, and teen rest needs
- Adjusting habits for adulthood and older age
- Family routines that respect everyone's rest

CHAPTER 17: HELPFUL TOOLS AND GADGETS

- Mattresses, pillows, and white noise devices
- Apps and trackers: benefits vs. risks
- Using tech wisely without adding stress

CHAPTER 18: SLEEPING AWAY FROM HOME

- Hotel tips, guest rooms, and camping basics
- Managing jet lag and unfamiliar beds
- Keeping a steady routine while traveling

CHAPTER 19: PUTTING IT ALL TOGETHER

- Combining daytime and nighttime strategies
- Building a personal plan and handling setbacks
- Tracking progress and staying flexible

CHAPTER 20: MAINTAINING PROGRESS

- Adapting when life changes affect rest
- Keeping motivation high over time
- Ensuring your good habits last for the future

Chapter 1: The Basics of Sleep

Sleep is one of the most important parts of our daily lives, yet many people do not know what sleep really does for the body and mind. It is not just a period of stillness. It is a time when the body carries out many tasks that help us stay healthy and ready for the next day. If you want to sleep better at night, it helps to begin with a clear look at what sleep really is and why it matters so much.

What is Sleep?

Sleep is a natural state of rest. During this time, the body rests, the mind sorts through memories, and cells repair themselves. Breathing and heart rate often slow down a bit. Different parts of the brain become more or less active. Even though the body looks inactive, a lot is going on inside.

People and many animals need sleep in order to survive. Lack of rest leads to problems with mood, memory, and even movement. Over time, poor sleep can raise the risk of health issues such as high blood pressure or problems with blood sugar. By knowing that sleep is not just "time off," we can start to treat it with more care.

Why Sleep is Important

1. **Memory and Learning**: While resting, the brain organizes and stores information. People who get enough rest often remember facts and details better than those who do not.
2. **Physical Health**: Muscle tissues repair themselves. The body makes certain hormones that help with growth and repair.
3. **Mood**: People who sleep well are more likely to feel calmer and patient. A lack of rest can cause crankiness, sadness, or worry.
4. **Energy**: Good sleep can help you feel more energetic during the day. You might find it easier to move around and focus on tasks.

Early Observations of Sleep

People have been trying to figure out sleep for a long time. Ancient cultures thought that the mind traveled to other places or that sleep was a state of quiet reflection. Later, scientists started to study sleep more closely. They watched how people breathed, checked their heart rates, and tracked brain waves. These studies taught us that sleep is a highly structured process that goes in cycles.

What Happens During Sleep

When you rest, the body goes through several states of sleep, which we will explore in the next chapter. In short, sleep states each have a different purpose. Some are more restful for the body, while others are more active for the mind. If these states are cut short, a person might wake up without feeling refreshed.

Daytime Activities That Affect Sleep

It is important to know that your daily habits can have a big effect on how you rest at night. Many people think of sleep as an event that happens only at bedtime, but it is actually linked to what we do during the day. Here are some factors:

- **Work and Study**: If a person has a lot of stress or tension from work or school, it can lead to restless nights. The brain stays active. It can be hard to relax.
- **Meal Times**: Eating very late or having large, heavy meals before bed can upset digestion and make it hard to fall asleep.
- **Substances**: Drinks that contain caffeine can keep you awake. Some medicines also interfere with rest.
- **Activity Level**: People who move around a lot during the day often find it easier to sleep at night.

Patterns from Childhood to Adulthood

Infants can sleep for most of the day, while older adults may rise early and go to bed early. Teenagers might stay up late and sleep in later. These patterns are not just due to habits. They are related to changes in our internal clocks and hormone release. Learning about these changes helps us understand why different age groups have different sleep patterns.

Short-Term Effects of Not Sleeping Well

A single night of poor rest can cause next-day problems. You might have trouble focusing on simple tasks. You might feel more annoyed by small things. Driving can be more dangerous because your reaction time slows down.

Some people think that losing a few hours of rest now and then is harmless, but it can add up. For example, a few nights of four or five hours of rest can lead to the same lack of focus and slowed reaction time as being awake for 24 hours straight. It is easy to see why making sleep a priority is so important.

Long-Term Effects of Not Sleeping Well

When bad sleep becomes a habit, serious problems may arise. Memory might fade. It can become harder to solve problems or to come up with new ideas. The immune system can weaken, making it easier to get sick. Also, the risk of health issues like heart disease and weight gain goes up.

Lack of rest also affects mood. Over time, it can lead to ongoing sadness or stress. It can even affect relationships, because a person might feel too tired to spend time with family and friends.

Signs You Might Need Better Rest

Many people do not realize their sleep is poor. They might think it is normal to feel groggy in the morning or to need an alarm clock just to get out of bed on time. Here are some signs that a person might need better rest:

1. Waking up feeling unready for the day.
2. Struggling to stay alert during tasks like reading or watching TV.
3. Frequent mood swings.
4. Needing naps too often to get through the day.
5. Difficulty remembering details or making quick decisions.

If these signs sound familiar, it might be time to look at your sleep habits and see if changes can be made.

Sleep: A Key Piece of Overall Health

Some people talk about diet and movement as top ways to stay healthy, but sleep is just as important. In fact, rest affects how you use food for energy and how well you respond to exercise. If you do not get enough rest, your body might react poorly to sugar and fat. Also, you might feel too tired to get active, which can lead to a cycle of low energy and poor health choices.

Simple Ways to Start Improving Sleep

1. **Set a Regular Bedtime**: The body likes routine. If you go to bed and get up at the same times, your internal clock starts to adjust.
2. **Avoid Screens**: Bright screens from phones or tablets can trick the brain into thinking it is still daytime. Reduce screen time an hour before bed.
3. **Watch What You Drink**: Limit caffeine to the early part of the day. Drinking too much in the afternoon can keep you awake.
4. **Make Your Bedroom Relaxing**: A cool, dark, and quiet room can help you fall asleep faster.
5. **Be Active During the Day**: Regular movement helps the body get tired at the right times.

Less-Known Tips for Better Rest

- **Ear Massage**: Some people find that gently rubbing the outer edges of the ear can help them relax. This simple act can calm the nervous system and prepare the body for sleep.
- **Foot Warmth**: Cold feet might keep you awake. Wearing socks or using a hot water bottle can help you rest more easily.
- **Breathing Patterns**: Inhaling for four seconds, holding for four seconds, and exhaling for four seconds can have a calming effect on the mind. This type of breathing can help slow the heart rate and reduce racing thoughts.
- **Hand Placement**: Placing a hand on the lower abdomen and noticing the rise and fall can help you stay present. This might slow mental chatter and guide you toward rest.

Changing Attitudes About Sleep

Many people see rest as something that gets in the way of productivity. They might stay up late to do more work or watch more shows. However, when we start to see sleep as an active part of staying healthy, we may adjust our schedules to fit in more rest.

Instead of thinking that a shorter night's sleep gives you more time, try looking at how much time is lost the next day because of feeling tired, unwell, or unable to focus. A well-rested mind can get more done in fewer hours because it is sharp and ready.

Cultural Differences in Sleep

In some places, taking midday rests or short breaks is common. In other cultures, people might frown on napping. Some cultures even have rules about bedtime for children. By learning from how different societies deal with rest, we can find what works best in our own lives.

Sleep is Personal

Not everyone needs the same amount of sleep. Some adults are fine on seven hours, while others need nine. The key is finding how many hours help you feel calm and focused. That can also change as you get older or go through big life events such as starting a new job or experiencing a major change in your family.

The Goal of This Book

We will look at many areas related to sleep. We will explore the different stages of rest, common sleep problems, stress, the bedroom environment, technology, nutrition, and more. Each chapter will give you clear facts and special tips you can use to improve your rest.

By the end of this book, you should have a good understanding of how sleep works, why it matters, and how to make adjustments that can help you sleep well each night. Whether you have trouble getting to sleep, staying asleep, or waking up feeling sluggish, the tips in this book can help you.

Small Action Steps

1. **Write a Sleep Diary**: For the next few days, write down when you went to bed, when you woke up, and how you felt. Look for patterns.
2. **Track Caffeine**: Note the times you drink coffee, tea, or other caffeinated drinks. See if you can cut back or drink them earlier in the day.
3. **Plan a Bedtime Activity**: Choose something relaxing, like reading a few pages of a book or listening to soft music. This can signal your brain that it is time to wind down.

These basic steps can pave the way for deeper improvements. In the next chapter, we will learn about the different stages of sleep and why each stage is important. That knowledge will help you see how a full cycle of rest can affect the way you feel when you open your eyes in the morning.

Chapter 2: Understanding Sleep Stages

In the last chapter, we looked at the basics of rest and why it matters. Now we will explore something a bit more specific: the different stages of sleep. Sleep might look like one long event, but it is actually made up of repeating cycles. Each cycle has separate stages. Understanding how they work can help you see why certain sleep problems happen and why some methods can help fix them.

Why Know About Sleep Stages?

When a person sleeps, the body goes through different levels of rest. Each level does something special. For instance, one stage might help with muscle repair, while another helps the brain process information from the day. If you often miss out on a certain stage—maybe because you are waking up often—you might feel specific problems. By learning about these stages, you can figure out better ways to help your body.

The Major Sleep Stages

Experts often place sleep into two main types: **Non-REM** (non-rapid eye movement) and **REM** (rapid eye movement). Non-REM sleep is broken into three stages:

1. **Stage N1 (Non-REM 1)**: This is the lightest form of sleep. During this stage, the person can be woken up easily. You might feel drowsy but still aware of your surroundings. The muscles might twitch. Some people also feel as if they are falling.
2. **Stage N2 (Non-REM 2)**: In this stage, the body relaxes more. Heart rate and breathing slow down a bit. Brain activity patterns shift to show that the body is settling in for deeper rest. You are less likely to be woken up by small noises.
3. **Stage N3 (Non-REM 3)**: This is a deep sleep stage. Breathing and heart rate reach their lowest levels, and brain waves slow down. It is hard to wake someone in this stage. If they do wake, they might feel groggy for a few minutes.

After spending time in these Non-REM stages, the body moves into REM sleep:

- **REM (Rapid Eye Movement) Sleep**: During this stage, the eyes move quickly under the eyelids, and brain activity looks quite similar to being awake. Most dreaming happens in this stage. Muscles in the arms and legs become briefly inactive, possibly to keep the body from acting out dreams.

Cycle Repeats

The sleep cycle typically repeats every 90 to 110 minutes. A person moves from the lighter stages to deeper stages and then into REM. Over the night, the amount of time spent in each stage changes. Early cycles often have longer deep sleep (N3). Toward morning, the body has more REM. This is why a person might recall vivid dreams when they wake up in the morning.

Deep Sleep: A Key Time for the Body

Deep sleep (stage N3) is also called slow-wave sleep. In this stage, the body repairs muscles and tissues. Energy is restored, and the immune system is strengthened. This is the part of sleep that makes you feel refreshed when you get out of bed. Missing out on deep sleep can lead to feeling physically tired.

Certain hormones, such as those related to growth, are also released in deeper sleep. In children and teens, these hormones help the body grow. In adults, they help with repair and upkeep of tissues.

REM Sleep: A Key Time for the Mind

REM is closely linked to memory and mood. The brain sorts through the day's experiences and decides what to keep or let go. It might even help with problem-solving. Some experts think that dreams help us handle emotions or set new ideas in our minds.

If you often wake up and never reach REM, you might find it harder to remember certain details. You might also experience changes in mood. Lack of REM has been linked to feeling low or stressed.

Changes with Age

Babies spend a lot of time in REM sleep, possibly because their brains are growing so fast. Older adults might have less time in deep sleep (N3) and more time in lighter stages. This can be why some older people wake up more at night or feel less rested in the morning. Children and teenagers might have strong deep sleep cycles, but they can also shift their sleep schedule, staying up late and sleeping in, which can affect how often they enter REM.

Outside Factors That Affect Stages

Many things can affect how the body moves through the sleep stages:

1. **Alcohol**: Drinking alcohol before bed can shorten REM and cause awakenings.
2. **Caffeine**: Taking caffeine too late in the day can prevent deep sleep.
3. **Drugs or Medications**: Certain medications change how much time is spent in each stage.
4. **Stress**: Worry can make it harder to drift into deeper stages. The mind stays alert, preventing you from dropping into a fully relaxed state.

Special Insights on Each Stage

Let's look closer at each sleep stage to see why it is special.

- **Stage N1**: Some might write this off as "barely sleeping," but it can be important because it helps the body move out of wakefulness. This is also a time when certain ideas or creative solutions pop up because the mind is relaxed but not fully shut off.
- **Stage N2**: This is the stage where you spend most of the night, as about half of total sleep time is in N2. Although it is not as deep as N3, it sets the stage for deeper rest. If you have trouble staying asleep, you might bounce back to N1 from N2, which can keep you from deeper levels.
- **Stage N3**: Deep sleep is often considered the most refreshing for the body. Some children have trouble waking up during this stage, or they might sleepwalk because the body is in a deep rest but the motor functions can still activate in odd ways.
- **REM**: In addition to dreaming, REM might help store memories more effectively. If you are working on a new skill, the brain could run through

that skill during REM to reinforce it. That is one reason well-rested people can learn new tasks more quickly.

Why You Might Not Get Enough of a Certain Stage

Some people have conditions that affect certain stages of sleep. For example:

- **Sleep Apnea**: When breathing stops for short periods, a person often wakes up enough to fix their breathing. This can prevent deep sleep and REM from happening enough.
- **Restless Leg Issues**: If a person's legs feel strange or they have an urge to move them, they might wake or move to a lighter stage.
- **Anxiety**: Racing thoughts might keep a person in lighter sleep. Their body stays on alert.

When a person does not get enough deep sleep, they might wake up with muscle aches. When a person does not get enough REM, they might feel mentally foggy or sad.

How to Support Each Stage

1. **Decrease Late-Day Stimulants**: Keeping caffeine in the early part of the day helps the body move into N3 more easily.
2. **Set a Regular Bedtime and Wake Time**: Going to bed and rising at the same times helps the body keep a predictable cycle.
3. **Manage Stress**: Relaxation methods and calm evening activities help the body settle into deeper stages.
4. **Limit Heavy Meals or Alcohol Close to Bed**: Alcohol might help you fall asleep fast, but it can disrupt later stages of rest. Heavy meals can cause digestion problems that keep you out of deep sleep.
5. **Physical Activity**: People who do moderate physical activity often experience better deep sleep. However, try not to exercise too close to bedtime because the body might be too energized to relax.

Special Tips to Strengthen Deep Sleep

- **Slow, Rhythmic Breathing Practice**: Before bed, do a few minutes of slow breathing. This helps lower the heart rate and can lead to deeper stages of rest.

- **Warm Bath**: Taking a warm bath an hour or two before bed can raise your body temperature. Once you leave the bath, your body begins to cool down, which signals the brain that it is time to rest.
- **Gentle Stretching**: Light stretches can help the muscles release tension. This can make it easier for the body to drop into deep sleep.

Special Tips to Strengthen REM Sleep

- **Balanced Light Exposure**: Getting enough daylight in the morning helps the body keep a stable internal clock. This stability allows a normal shift from deep sleep to REM at night.
- **Avoid Going to Bed with Intense Worries**: If you are thinking about big concerns, you might experience less restful REM. Writing down thoughts or simple lists of solutions can help calm the mind.
- **Sleep Enough Hours**: REM periods get longer toward morning. If you cut your sleep short by waking up too early, you might lose REM cycles.

Dream Recall and Emotional Health

Some people remember their dreams, while others do not. It depends on when you wake up and how your brain stores memories. Sometimes, recalling dreams can give hints about emotional or mental states. If dreams are often scary, it might point to high stress or unresolved worries. While you do not have to analyze every dream, noticing patterns can help you see if something is bothering you.

Tech Tools for Tracking Sleep Stages

Many modern devices can track sleep patterns. Wristbands, phone apps, and special mattresses can measure movement or heart rate and give you an idea of how long you spend in each stage. While these devices are not perfect, they can offer clues. If you see that you are getting a lot of light sleep but little deep or REM sleep, you can make changes based on the tips above.

However, keep in mind that these tools can sometimes cause extra worry. If you get too focused on the numbers, you might end up feeling anxious, which can hurt your rest. Use them as guides, not strict judges.

Setting Realistic Goals

It might be tempting to try to force more deep sleep or REM time right away. But the best approach is often to aim for a healthy routine that allows your body to do its work. A good routine includes going to bed at a time that fits your schedule, waking up at a regular time, keeping the bedroom comfortable, and making smart choices about substances like caffeine and alcohol.

Over time, you might notice you feel more refreshed in the morning. That can be a sign you are getting more deep sleep. You might also recall more dreams or find it easier to handle emotional ups and downs, showing you are getting healthy REM cycles.

Common Misconceptions About Sleep Stages

1. **"I Only Need One Sleep Cycle."** Some claim a single cycle of 90 minutes is enough, but this is not true for most people. We need several cycles to get enough deep and REM sleep.
2. **"I Can Make Up All Lost Sleep in One Weekend."** Catching up on rest might help a bit, but it may not fully fix weeks of poor sleep. Also, sleeping late on weekends can shift your body clock, making it harder to fall asleep on Sunday night.
3. **"I Woke Up Right After a Dream, So I Did Not Get Any Deep Sleep."** Not true. We shift through stages multiple times. Waking after a dream could just mean you were in REM at that moment.

When to See a Professional

If you try basic tips but still wake up feeling unready for the day, it might be wise to see a sleep specialist. There are tests like the polysomnogram that measure brain waves, breathing, and muscle activity as you rest. A specialist can see if you have a disorder like sleep apnea or restless leg syndrome and can suggest treatments.

Some clues you might need professional help include:

- Loud snoring or gasping for air.
- Frequent waking with a racing heart.
- Persistent feeling of sadness or worry that keeps you from sleeping.

- Strange behaviors during the night like sleepwalking that put you or others at risk.

Gaining Control Over Your Night

Many people think they have little control over how they sleep, but that is not always true. We can guide our habits, manage our stress, and adjust our environment. The process might take time, but by steadily making changes, we can shape our sleep stages in a more helpful way.

Little-Known Ways to Improve Stage Quality

- **Listening to Soft Rhythms**: Light, repetitive sounds can help the brain settle into a calm pattern. This could be gentle music or nature sounds.
- **Cooling the Room**: The body temperature needs to drop slightly to fall asleep. A cooler room can help the brain enter deeper sleep faster.
- **Early Bright Light**: Spending time in the morning sunlight helps regulate the internal clock, ensuring that you get a proper REM cycle at night.

In Summary

Sleep is divided into different stages, each playing a role in mind and body health. Deep sleep helps fix tissues and renew energy. REM helps with learning, memory, and mood. The body cycles through these stages multiple times per night, and different things can affect how much time you spend in each stage. Knowing about these stages can guide you toward better habits, routines, and choices.

In the next chapters, we will look at common sleep problems and how stress ties into the rest you get. The more you understand about each aspect of rest, the easier it becomes to spot simple changes that can make a big difference.

Quick Suggestions to Start Applying

1. **Keep a Regular Bedtime**: This helps the body's internal clock so you move through stages in the right order.
2. **Reduce Late Night Distractions**: Lights, noises, and screens can prevent you from slipping into deeper rest.

3. **Try Gentle Wind-Down Techniques**: Relax your body and mind before bed so you can reach deeper stages sooner.
4. **Check Your Room Temperature**: A cool room is often best for sleep cycles.

By understanding sleep stages, you can start to see that rest is not just "on" or "off." It is a detailed process that moves through different states. Each state helps you in a special way, from building muscle to sorting your memories. This knowledge can help you address specific sleep problems. If you often feel tired in the morning or have trouble focusing, it might be that your sleep stages are being cut short. And when you know why, you can work on things that will help you get the rest you need.

Chapter 3: Common Sleep Problems

In the previous chapters, we learned about the basics of rest and the stages that our bodies move through each night. Now, we will focus on different problems that can arise when trying to sleep. These problems affect people all around the world and can make it very hard to feel refreshed in the morning. While some of these issues can be minor and happen only once in a while, others might need special care. By learning about the different types of sleep problems, their signs, and possible fixes, you can catch them early and find ways to improve your rest.

1. Insomnia

Overview
Insomnia is one of the most common sleep problems. It involves difficulty falling asleep, staying asleep, or both. Some people with insomnia wake up too early and find they cannot fall back to sleep. Others lie awake for a long time before drifting off. When insomnia lasts for only a few days or weeks, it is often called short-term insomnia. When it becomes a regular problem for months, it is known as long-term insomnia.

Possible Causes

- Stress about work, school, finances, or personal events.
- Irregular sleep schedule, such as frequently changing bedtimes.
- Consuming caffeine late in the day.
- A noisy or uncomfortable bedroom.
- Ongoing worry or mood problems.

Signs

- Lying awake for more than 30 minutes when trying to sleep.
- Waking up many times during the night.
- Feeling tired or irritated during the day.
- Relying on naps or stimulants (like coffee) to get through the day.

Less-Known Facts

- Bright lights from screens and overhead bulbs can lower the body's natural production of certain hormones that help you sleep.
- Some people with insomnia have a hard time sensing when their bodies are actually relaxed. Their minds keep running, so they assume they are still awake, even when they might be lightly dozing off.

Ways to Handle Insomnia

- **Set a Stable Schedule**: Go to bed and wake up at the same times every day, even on weekends.
- **Practice Calm Thoughts**: Some people try a simple counting method or focus on a single mental image to keep racing thoughts away.
- **Limit Screen Time**: Reducing screen use in the hour before bed can help.
- **Limit Naps**: If you must nap, keep it brief, around 20-30 minutes, and not too close to bedtime.
- **Speak with a Professional**: If insomnia becomes severe, a therapist or doctor can help.

---

2. Sleep Apnea

Overview

Sleep apnea is a condition that involves short pauses in breathing while sleeping. During these pauses, a person might snore or snort, then suddenly start breathing again. This disrupts the normal flow of sleep stages, often preventing the body from reaching deep sleep and REM. There are two main types:

- **Obstructive Sleep Apnea (OSA)**: Caused by a blockage in the airway, often due to relaxed throat muscles or extra tissue around the neck.
- **Central Sleep Apnea (CSA)**: The brain does not send the right signals to the muscles that control breathing.

Possible Causes

- Having a thicker neck circumference or extra weight around the neck.
- Relaxed throat muscles during sleep.
- Certain physical features, like a narrow airway.

- Advanced age or certain health problems (for CSA).

Signs

- Loud snoring, often followed by a moment of silence, then a sudden gasp or snort.
- Feeling tired in the morning even after a full night in bed.
- Morning headaches or a dry mouth.
- Mood or focus problems during the day.

Less-Known Facts

- People with sleep apnea might wake up dozens or even hundreds of times each night. These interruptions can be so brief that the person does not recall them.
- Certain sleeping positions can increase or decrease breathing problems. Some individuals with OSA find it easier to breathe on their sides rather than their back.

Ways to Handle Sleep Apnea

- **Lifestyle Changes**: Losing some weight, improving fitness, and avoiding alcohol close to bedtime can lower apnea episodes.
- **Positional Therapy**: Some use special devices to keep them from rolling onto their backs.
- **CPAP Machine**: A mask worn during sleep delivers constant air pressure, keeping the airway open.
- **Oral Appliances**: Dental devices can hold the jaw forward to prevent the tongue from blocking the airway.
- **Medical Procedures**: In some cases, surgery can remove extra tissue or change the shape of the airway.

---

3. Restless Legs and Other Movement Issues

Overview

Some people feel a strong urge to move their legs at night. This is often called Restless Legs issues. They might also feel a crawling or tingling feeling in the calves or thighs. Movement can help briefly, but the urge often returns when they stop moving.

Possible Causes

- Low iron levels in the body.
- Certain medical conditions, such as kidney issues or diabetes.
- Pregnancy can trigger these symptoms for some individuals.
- Nerve problems or side effects from certain medications.

Signs

- Uncomfortable sensations in the legs when resting.
- Feeling better only when walking or stretching.
- Trouble settling down in bed due to these sensations.

Less-Known Facts

- Some people may experience similar urges in their arms, although it is much rarer.
- The condition can become worse with stress or a lack of certain minerals in the diet.

Ways to Handle Restless Legs

- **Check Iron Levels**: A simple blood test can reveal if you have low iron.
- **Avoid Caffeine and Alcohol**: Both can worsen the sensations.
- **Try Warm or Cool Packs**: Applying heat or cold can soothe the limbs.
- **Light Stretches**: Gentle movements of the legs before bedtime might reduce symptoms.

---

4. Narcolepsy

Overview

Narcolepsy is a condition that causes too much daytime sleepiness. People with narcolepsy can fall asleep suddenly and without warning. These episodes might happen during normal daily activities, like having a conversation or eating a meal. It can be dangerous if it happens while driving or handling machinery.

Possible Causes

- A lower level of a chemical in the brain that helps control wakefulness.
- Sometimes triggered by infections or immune system responses.
- Can run in families, though not always.

Signs

- Sudden "sleep attacks" during the day.
- Cataplexy: a sudden weakness in the muscles, often triggered by strong emotions like laughter or surprise.
- Fragmented nighttime sleep, with multiple awakenings.

Less-Known Facts

- People with narcolepsy can experience vivid dreams at the start of sleep or right upon waking.
- Narcolepsy is rare but often misunderstood. Some think those with narcolepsy are just lazy, which is not accurate.

Ways to Handle Narcolepsy

- **Medication**: Certain stimulants or alertness-boosting drugs can help manage daytime sleepiness.
- **Scheduled Naps**: Brief rests during the day can help control sudden sleep episodes.
- **Lifestyle Adjustments**: Avoiding heavy meals and alcohol can reduce daytime fatigue.

---

5. Circadian Rhythm Disorders

Overview

Our bodies have internal clocks that guide when we feel awake and when we feel tired. When this clock gets out of sync, we call it a circadian rhythm disorder. One example is "Delayed Sleep Phase," where a person naturally falls asleep very late and wakes up late. Another is "Advanced Sleep Phase," where a person is sleepy early in the evening and wakes up too early.

Possible Causes

- Irregular work schedules, like rotating shifts.
- Traveling across multiple time zones (jet lag).
- Hormonal shifts, especially in teenagers.
- Lack of morning sunlight.

Signs

- Finding it hard to fall asleep at normal times.
- Feeling wide awake late into the night or too early in the morning.
- Feeling out of sync with local schedules, especially after travel.

Less-Known Facts

- The body's clock is slightly longer than 24 hours for most people. Sunlight each morning helps reset it.
- Teenagers tend to have a delayed clock naturally, which can clash with early school start times.

Ways to Handle Circadian Rhythm Disorders

- **Light Exposure**: Morning sunlight or light therapy boxes can help shift the clock earlier.
- **Controlled Melatonin**: Under a doctor's advice, small doses at certain times might help reset the rhythm.
- **Consistent Schedule**: Going to sleep and waking up at the same times each day can reinforce your body's clock.

---

6. Nightmares and Other Disturbing Dreams

Overview

Most of us have upsetting dreams sometimes, but if nightmares occur often, they can disrupt sleep. They may be linked to real events in daily life, or they might have no obvious trigger. Nightmares are more common in children but can also happen in adults.

Possible Causes

- Stressful experiences or trauma.
- Watching scary or disturbing content before bed.
- Some medications.
- Eating heavy meals close to bedtime (can lead to more intense dreams).

Signs

- Waking up with clear recall of a disturbing dream.
- Feeling anxious about going to sleep for fear of having another nightmare.
- Trouble falling asleep again after a nightmare.

Less-Known Facts

- Adults sometimes have nightmares that are tied to major life changes or intense worries they have not faced while awake.
- Repeated nightmares about the same theme might signal ongoing stress that needs addressing.

Ways to Handle Nightmares

- **Soothing Bedtime Routine**: Practice a calming activity.
- **Avoid Scary Content**: This includes movies or shows before bed.
- **Jot Down Worries**: Writing them on paper might reduce their power at night.
- **Seek Help**: If nightmares stem from deep emotional or mental issues, counseling can help.

---

7. Teeth Grinding (Bruxism)

Overview

Teeth grinding or clenching can happen at night without a person even knowing. Over time, this can lead to tooth damage, jaw pain, and disrupted sleep.

Possible Causes

- Stress or worry.

- An abnormal bite or missing teeth.
- Certain sleep disorders like apnea can increase the chance of grinding.

Signs

- Waking up with a sore jaw, ears, or head.
- A partner hearing clicking or grinding noises at night.
- Teeth appearing worn or chipped.

Less-Known Facts

- Some people hold stress in their jaw muscles, which can carry over into sleep.
- Teeth grinding can sometimes be linked to heartburn or acid reflux, though not as commonly.

Ways to Handle Bruxism

- **Mouth Guard**: A custom-fitted guard can reduce pressure on the teeth.
- **Stress Control**: Relaxation steps can help those who grind due to tension.
- **Jaw Exercises**: Some specialists recommend simple exercises to loosen the jaw.

---

8. Parasomnias (Odd Actions During Sleep)

Overview
Parasomnias are unusual movements or behaviors that happen during sleep. These can include sleepwalking, talking in sleep, eating during the night without remembering, or even more complex actions.

Possible Causes

- Partial awakenings during deep sleep.
- Family history of parasomnias.
- Disruption of the normal sleep cycle, such as from stress or irregular schedules.

Signs

- Doing things at night that you do not recall in the morning.
- Having a partner or family member notice odd behaviors.
- Waking up in different parts of the house without knowing how you got there.

Less-Known Facts

- Some sleepwalkers go through a detailed routine, like getting dressed or leaving the house.
- Night terrors are a type of parasomnia common in children. During these episodes, a child might scream or seem panicked but have no memory of it the next day.

Ways to Handle Parasomnias

- **Improve Safety**: Lock doors and remove sharp or dangerous objects.
- **Check Medications**: Some prescriptions can trigger these episodes.
- **Sleep Study**: A professional test can see if there is an underlying issue like apnea.

---

9. Shift Work Sleep Problems

Overview
People who work at night or rotate their schedules face a high risk of disturbed sleep. This problem comes from having to be awake when it is dark and sleeping when it is light, which goes against the body's natural rhythm.

Possible Causes

- Inconsistent work hours.
- Bright daylight exposure when trying to sleep.
- Drinking coffee or energy drinks to stay awake at work.

Signs

- Struggling to fall asleep during the daytime.

- Feeling tired during night shifts.
- Changes in mood and focus.

Less-Known Facts

- Many industrial accidents have been linked to tired workers on night shifts.
- Some people manage shift work better than others because of differences in their body clocks.

Ways to Handle Shift Work Problems

- **Limit Morning Sunlight After Work**: Wear sunglasses on your way home so your body does not "wake up" too much.
- **Establish a Dark Sleeping Space**: Use blackout curtains or eye masks.
- **Stick to a Schedule**: Even on days off, try not to switch too drastically to a normal daytime rhythm.
- **Use Artificial Light Wisely**: When waking up for a night shift, bright light can help signal your body to become alert.

---

10. Unusual Conditions

There are some other rare conditions that can affect a person's rest. These might include:

- **Sleep Paralysis**: Being briefly unable to move or speak right after waking or before falling asleep.
- **Hallucinations**: Some people see or hear things that are not there during the transition between waking and sleeping.
- **Catathrenia**: Making long moaning or groaning sounds during exhalation in the night.

Possible Causes

- Disruptions in the normal sleep-wake cycle.
- Stress or trauma.
- Certain neurological conditions.

Signs

- Brief confusion upon waking.
- Feeling panic during episodes.
- Partners or roommates noticing the noises or behaviors.

Less-Known Facts

- Sleep paralysis can feel frightening, but it is usually harmless and lasts only a short time.
- Many of these conditions improve when a person adopts healthier sleep patterns.

Ways to Handle Unusual Conditions

- **Reassurance**: Learning that these states are usually not dangerous can reduce fear.
- **Better Sleep Habits**: A consistent bedtime, lowered stress, and limited screen time can ease these states.
- **Professional Evaluation**: If these conditions happen often and cause distress, a doctor might suggest a sleep study.

Why Early Detection Matters

Spotting a sleep problem early on can prevent larger health issues. Sometimes a small adjustment in habits or environment is all that is needed to fix a problem. Other times, medical support might be required. Either way, ignoring ongoing sleep problems can lead to serious effects on mood, alertness, and long-term health. For example, untreated apnea can raise blood pressure or add strain on the heart. Chronic insomnia can lead to sadness or worry disorders. By recognizing signs and seeking solutions, people can address these concerns head-on.

When to Seek Professional Help

Not all sleep issues can be fixed on your own. If you notice any of these, it might be time to see a specialist:

- You regularly wake up gasping for air or have been told that you stop breathing at night.
- You feel so tired during the day that it affects your work, school, or social life.
- You have severe or disturbing behaviors at night, such as episodes of sleepwalking that put you at risk.
- Your moods or mental health have taken a downturn because of poor rest.
- You have tried self-help methods for a long time without improvement.

Sleep professionals might run tests such as a polysomnogram, which measures breathing, brain waves, and muscle activity during rest. They could also suggest treatments for any underlying medical issues.

Special Measures and Tools

Mouthguards
These devices help people with snoring or teeth grinding. They can be custom-made by a dentist or purchased over the counter, though a custom fit is often better.

Apps and Wearables
While the accuracy can vary, some phone apps and wrist gadgets track movement, heart rate, and even oxygen levels. These might give you clues about how often you wake up or how much you move in your sleep. However, keep in mind that these are not always 100% accurate.

Medication
For some conditions, short-term or long-term medication can help. For example, people with narcolepsy might take stimulants to avoid daytime episodes. Those with restless legs might need a specific drug that helps soothe the sensations.

Therapy

Cognitive methods can help those with insomnia change their thinking patterns. For nightmares, some mental techniques teach a person to rewrite the ending of a bad dream in their mind while awake, reducing its negative effects.

Putting This Knowledge to Use

If you think you might have one of these problems, try these steps:

1. **Record Your Symptoms**: Note when the problem started, how often it happens, and what your nights are like.
2. **Check Your Habits**: See if you are using screens late, drinking too much caffeine, or sleeping in an environment that is not quiet or dark.
3. **Try Simple Changes First**: Adjust your routine, make your bedroom calmer, and watch what you eat or drink in the evening.
4. **Reach Out for Guidance**: If self-help steps do not work, a doctor or therapist can guide you further.

Understanding these problems and taking action early can help keep them from getting worse. Whether the problem is insomnia, sleep apnea, or an unusual behavior at night, many solutions are available. It might feel frustrating at times, but making the right changes can help you start to feel better.

Chapter Summary

Common sleep problems include insomnia, apnea, restless legs, narcolepsy, circadian rhythm issues, nightmares, and more. Each has specific signs and causes, but all can affect how refreshed you feel each day. Some, like insomnia, might be eased by improving habits and routines. Others, like apnea, may need medical tools or procedures. No matter what the issue is, early recognition, a willingness to make changes, and seeking help when needed can lead to better sleep. In the next chapter, we will look at how stress ties into rest, because stress can make existing sleep problems worse or even spark new ones.

Chapter 4: The Link Between Sleep and Stress

We have covered different sleep problems that can affect a person's ability to get a good night's rest. One of the biggest factors that can cause or worsen these problems is stress. Stress is a normal response to the demands of everyday life, but when it becomes constant, it can put the body and mind under pressure. This can lead to poor sleep, which in turn can increase stress. It can become a cycle that is hard to break. In this chapter, we will look at how stress and rest affect each other. We will also discuss some techniques and lesser-known tips to manage stress for better rest.

1. What is Stress?

Stress can be described as the body's reaction to threats or challenges. It triggers changes in the body, such as a faster heart rate and higher blood pressure. The goal of this reaction is to prepare us to face or get away from the source of stress. This process is often referred to as the "fight or flight" response. While a little stress can help motivate us, too much can harm our well-being and reduce our ability to sleep.

2. How Stress Disrupts Sleep

Elevated Heart Rate

When you are stressed, your body stays on alert. Heart rate remains higher than normal, and the body produces chemicals that prevent it from fully relaxing. These chemicals might make it harder to drift into the deeper stages of rest.

Mind Racing

Stress often causes racing thoughts. You might lie in bed replaying events of the day or worrying about tasks you have to do in the future. Instead of drifting off, you remain caught in mental tension.

Interrupted Stages

Even if you manage to fall asleep, stress can lead to fragmented rest. You may shift from deep sleep to a lighter stage or wake up during the night because the mind is still partly active and on guard.

Increased Tension in Muscles

Stress causes the muscles to tighten, particularly in the shoulders, neck, or jaw. This tension can keep you from feeling comfortable in bed. It might also lead to physical aches that disrupt rest.

---

3. How Lack of Sleep Increases Stress

Just as stress can ruin your rest, poor sleep can also intensify stress. Here's how:

1. **Worse Mood**: Without enough rest, the brain might overreact to small issues. You can feel annoyed or upset more easily.
2. **Reduced Coping Skills**: When you are exhausted, it is harder to handle normal challenges. Tasks that would be simple when rested can seem overwhelming.
3. **Confusion and Worry**: Lack of sleep can affect memory and focus, which can cause you to worry about mistakes or forget important duties, adding more stress.

Over time, this can form a cycle: Stress harms rest, poor rest increases stress, and so forth.

---

4. The Role of Hormones

When discussing stress, two key chemicals come up: **cortisol** and **adrenaline**. Cortisol helps regulate how the body uses sugars and fats, and it also influences sleep-wake patterns. When under stress, cortisol can rise too high at night, making it difficult to relax. Adrenaline is released to help you handle an immediate threat, increasing heart rate and tightening muscles. If adrenaline stays high, it can cause trouble drifting off or staying asleep.

Less-Known Fact: Cortisol levels normally rise just before waking up in the morning, giving you energy to start the day. If these levels are disrupted by chronic stress, you might either feel wired at bedtime or lack energy at the time you actually need it.

---

5. Stress Triggers That Harm Sleep

- **Financial Problems**: Worrying about bills or debt.
- **Work Overload**: Tight deadlines or tough office dynamics.
- **Personal Conflicts**: Disagreements with friends or family.
- **Big Life Events**: Moves, job changes, or major personal losses.
- **Technology Overuse**: Constant messages or checking social media can stress the mind.

Though these triggers are common, each person might have additional ones. Recognizing personal triggers is the first step toward fixing them.

---

6. Physical Effects of Stress on the Body at Night

When you lie down to rest, you might think the body automatically relaxes. However, stress can cause several hidden reactions:

- **Raised Body Temperature**: Stress can prevent the body from cooling down, which is needed to start sleep.
- **Upset Digestion**: Some experience stomach issues when stressed, leading to discomfort in bed.
- **Rapid Breathing**: Shallow or fast breathing can disturb the calm needed for deeper rest.

These changes might not be obvious, but they play a large part in whether you get a solid night of rest.

---

7. Recognizing High Stress Levels

Sometimes, people do not realize they are under high stress until they struggle to sleep. Here are some signs:

- Feeling easily annoyed or impatient.
- Having trouble focusing during the day.
- Frequent headaches or tension in the neck.
- Gritting teeth or clenching jaw.
- Racing thoughts when trying to relax.

If several of these signs match your experience, it might indicate that your stress levels are too high.

8. Methods to Lower Stress for Better Sleep

1. **Breathing Techniques**
   - **4-4-4 Method**: Inhale through the nose for four seconds, hold the breath for four seconds, and exhale for four seconds. This pattern can signal to the body that it is safe to relax.
   - **Long Exhale**: Inhale for four seconds, but exhale for six or eight seconds. Longer exhalations can reduce tension in the nervous system.
2. **Progressive Muscle Relaxation**
   This involves tensing and then relaxing each muscle group in your body. Begin with the toes, then move up to the calves, thighs, abdomen, and so on until you reach the face. This practice can reduce stress-related tension.
3. **Thought Shifting**
   When thoughts start to swirl, try focusing on a neutral or simple image, like a gentle light or a quiet place. If a worry enters your mind, note it briefly, then return your focus to your chosen image.
4. **Writing It Down**
   Spend a few minutes before bed writing any tasks or worries. Placing them on paper can give your mind permission to let them rest until morning.
5. **Gentle Physical Activity**
   A short walk or some light stretching in the early evening can help lower built-up stress. Avoid intense exercise close to bedtime, as that might stimulate you more.
6. **Limit News Exposure at Night**
   Reading or watching stressful news in the evening can spike stress chemicals in the body. Try to stay informed earlier in the day instead.

9. Setting Boundaries

Many sources of stress involve other people or responsibilities. Setting personal boundaries can help. For example:

- **Work Boundaries**: If possible, avoid reading work emails after a certain hour.
- **Social Boundaries**: Gently let friends or family know that late-night calls or texts might interfere with rest.
- **Technology Boundaries**: Silence or keep devices away from the bedroom.

These steps can reduce late-evening stress triggers that make it hard to relax at night.

---

10. The Idea of "Worry Time"

Some people find it helpful to pick a specific time of day to think about or list their worries. This might sound strange, but it can help the mind avoid stress loops at bedtime. By giving yourself a daily "appointment" with your worries—say, 20 minutes in the late afternoon—you teach your brain that it does not need to chase these thoughts at night.

---

11. Stress, Food, and Sleep

Stress can alter your eating patterns. Some people lose appetite, while others overeat, often choosing sugary or fatty foods for comfort. Both extremes can harm your rest:

- **Too Little Food**: Going to bed hungry might cause late-night awakenings.
- **Too Heavy Meals**: Large dinners can cause heartburn or indigestion.
- **Sugary Snacks**: Can cause spikes in blood sugar, followed by crashes that disrupt sleep later.

Less-Known Fact: Some individuals with high stress have cravings for salty snacks, which can contribute to water retention and disturb the body's natural balance. Making steady food choices and watching portion sizes can help keep rest on track.

12. Stress and Hormone Release Timing

We mentioned earlier how cortisol and adrenaline can rise with stress. However, stress can also disrupt other hormones that promote rest, such as melatonin. If your body is too tense, it might delay or reduce melatonin production at night. As a result, you stay more alert than you should be.

Practical Tip: Getting morning sunlight helps set the timer for melatonin release at night. If you face high stress, a consistent morning routine that includes sunlight can help anchor your system.

---

13. The Connection Between Stress, Anxiety, and Sleep

Although "stress" and "anxiety" are not exactly the same, they often overlap. Chronic stress can turn into an anxiety problem if left unchecked. This, in turn, can further disrupt rest. You may experience muscle tension, rapid heartbeat, and intrusive thoughts.

Ways to Break the Cycle

- **Mindful Reading**: Read a calming book before bed rather than something intense.
- **Relaxing Sounds**: Gentle background noises, like soft nature sounds, can lower anxiety.
- **Steady Habits**: Regular sleep times and routines can give anxious minds a sense of predictability.

14. Work and School Stress

Our jobs and schoolwork are major sources of stress for many people. Deadlines, exams, or presentations can cause nighttime worry. Some might even dream about work or school conflicts, leading to restless nights.

Tips to Manage This Stress

- **Plan Ahead**: Write down tasks that need doing the next day before you end your current workday.

- **Divide Large Tasks**: Break big tasks into smaller parts that you can handle one at a time. This helps you feel less overwhelmed.
- **Find Small Wins**: Note small successes each day, so your mind ends on a positive note rather than a list of failures or undone tasks.

---

15. Family and Relationship Stress

Arguments and misunderstandings with loved ones can also disrupt rest. You might go to bed upset or worried about an unresolved fight. Such emotional distress can keep the body on high alert.

Ideas to Ease Relationship Stress

- **Clear Communication**: Try to talk through concerns earlier in the evening, not at bedtime.
- **Agree to Pause**: If you cannot resolve an issue, agree to pause the argument and revisit it calmly later, rather than staying up stewing over it.
- **Show Kindness**: Simple acts of kindness or apologies can reduce tension and help both sides relax before bedtime.

---

16. Unusual Stress Sources

Sometimes, stress does not come from the obvious things like finances or work. It could stem from deeper worries or hidden triggers. For example:

- **Background Noise**: A slight humming sound or dripping tap might annoy you and make you feel on edge without realizing why.
- **Mental Overstimulation**: Engaging with too many social media notifications can create a sense of constant mental chatter.
- **Fear of Missing Out**: Feeling pressured to do everything, see everyone, and never miss an event.

Identifying less obvious stress sources can help you remove them or manage them better.

17. Techniques for Quick Calm-Down

If you are in bed and realize you are feeling stressed, here are some quick tips:

1. **Hand Relaxation**: Slowly open and close your hands, focusing on the movement. This can distract from anxious thoughts.
2. **Warm Compress on the Eyes**: A gentle warm compress on the forehead or eyes can ease tension.
3. **Count Breaths Backward**: Count down from 50 or 100 with each breath. If you lose track, start again. The simple act of counting can be calming.

---

18. Creating a Stress-Free Evening Routine

A good evening routine can prevent stress from creeping into your nighttime hours. Consider steps such as:

- **Shut Down Work**: Have a firm cutoff time for work or study tasks.
- **Dim the Lights**: Lower the brightness around your home as bedtime approaches.
- **Calming Hobby**: A quiet hobby, like simple crafts or putting together a puzzle, can help calm the mind.
- **Low-Volume Music**: Soft tunes with slow tempo can help slow your heart rate.

Making these parts of your daily routine sets a clear signal to your mind that the day's active phase is ending.

---

19. Longer-Term Methods to Reduce Stress

Apart from the quick tips, there are some longer-term ways to address stress:

- **Therapy or Counseling**: A mental health professional can teach strategies to manage ongoing stress.
- **Physical Activity**: Regular moderate movement can burn off stress chemicals and increase calm feelings, though it should be done earlier in the day.

- **Mindful Awareness**: Being aware of what triggers you can help you avoid or manage situations more proactively.
- **Social Support**: Sharing your concerns with a friend or support group can help lighten the mental load.

20. Bringing It All Together

The link between stress and rest is strong. Stress causes the body and mind to remain on alert, making it harder to fall and stay asleep. Poor rest leads to higher stress the next day, fueling a cycle. By understanding how stress affects the body's chemistry, sleep stages, and mental state, we can act sooner to keep stress from harming our nights.

When you notice tension or worry creeping in, try a few simple actions: slow breathing, writing thoughts down, or putting away your phone. If your stress levels seem unmanageable, do not hesitate to talk to someone you trust or a health professional. Breaking the cycle of stress and poor rest can improve not only your nights but also your overall well-being.

Chapter Summary

Stress and rest are strongly linked. Stress triggers changes in the body that keep it from relaxing, leading to poor rest. Poor rest makes you feel tired, irritated, and worried the next day, creating a loop that can be hard to escape. Recognizing personal stress triggers, using simple relaxation methods, setting boundaries, and seeking help if needed can break this cycle. By taking specific steps—like using breathing techniques, setting a worry time, or adjusting your evening routine—you can lower stress and encourage a calm mind at night. In future chapters, we will look at more steps to build a good sleep environment, how technology and different lifestyle choices factor into rest, and ways to keep building on these improvements.

Chapter 5: Building a Good Sleep Environment

We have explored why rest matters and how stress, routines, and different problems affect your sleep. Now, it is time to look at the physical space where you rest. A bed is only part of the story. The entire room can either help you relax or make it harder to fall asleep. In this chapter, we will discuss how to set up your space in a way that helps your mind and body wind down each night. We will also offer lesser-known tips that can make a difference.

1. Why the Bedroom Matters

The place where you sleep has a big impact on the quality of your rest. A welcoming room can help you feel calm, while a messy or uninviting room can make it hard to relax. Think about how you feel when you go on a trip and sleep in a comfortable hotel room that is clean and quiet. You may find it easier to settle down. On the other hand, if you stay in a loud and hot place, you might toss and turn. By adjusting your space at home, you can create a similar calm feeling that signals rest.

2. Temperature and Air Quality

Optimal Temperature

Many people find that a room between about 60 to 68 degrees Fahrenheit (15.5 to 20 degrees Celsius) is comfortable. Of course, personal preference matters. Some sleep better when it is slightly warmer; others like it cooler. If the room is too hot, your body may sweat and your heart rate might stay elevated. If it is too cold, you might feel tense. Either extreme can interfere with deeper stages of rest.

Lesser-Known Tip: Having a warm bath or shower 60 to 90 minutes before bedtime can raise your core temperature slightly. Then, when you step out, your body begins to cool, which may help you fall asleep faster.

Humidity

If the air is very dry, you might experience a scratchy throat or dry skin. On the other hand, high humidity can cause sweating and discomfort. A moderate level of humidity, usually around 40 to 50 percent, can help you breathe easier. You can measure humidity using a small device called a hygrometer. If it is too high, use a dehumidifier. If it is too low, consider a humidifier.

Lesser-Known Tip: Some humidifiers allow you to add drops of mild, calming oils (like certain plant-based extracts). While strong smells can be overwhelming, a gentle scent might help your mind settle.

Air Circulation

Fresh air is important. If your room is stuffy, you may wake up with a blocked nose or slight headache. Opening a window briefly each day, if weather and noise levels allow, can refresh the room. If that is not possible, using a fan or air purifier can help move air around and filter out particles.

---

3. Light Levels

Natural Light in the Morning

Sunlight in the morning helps control your internal clock. If possible, let natural light into your room soon after you wake up. This can make it easier for your body to know it is daytime, which in turn sets the stage for better rest at night.

Darkness at Night

When it is time to sleep, darkness sends a signal to the brain that it is time to rest. Streetlights, hallway bulbs, or blue light from electronics can confuse the brain. Blackout curtains or blinds can help if you live in a bright area, or if you work night shifts and must sleep during the day. If you cannot block out all light, a sleep mask is a simpler option.

Lesser-Known Tip: Some people find that red-tinted night lights (instead of bright white ones) are less disruptive if they need to get up in the middle of the night. Red light has a lower impact on the body's natural signals.

4. Sound Control

Importance of Quiet

Noise disrupts rest. Even if you do not fully wake up, sounds can pull you out of deeper sleep stages. Over time, this might leave you feeling tired. Common sources of noise include traffic, neighbors, and even the humming of appliances.

Solutions

- **Earplugs**: A simple and affordable way to block out noise. Make sure they fit well and do not cause discomfort.
- **White Noise Machines**: Some devices create steady background sounds like rainfall or static. These can mask sudden noises.
- **Heavy Curtains or Carpets**: Thick materials help dampen sound that comes from outside or other rooms.

Lesser-Known Tip: If you struggle with random sounds at night, some apps or gadgets provide "pink noise" or "brown noise" as well, which some users find more soothing than plain white noise.

---

5. Furniture and Layout

Bed and Mattress

The bed should be supportive and match your comfort needs. A mattress that is too hard can cause pressure points, while one that is too soft might not support your spine. Pillows also matter. A good pillow keeps your head and neck in line with your spine. Some people prefer memory foam; others like a classic pillow. The key is feeling comfortable and well-aligned.

Position of the Bed

While there is no single correct spot for everyone, try to place your bed in a way that feels calm and secure. Many prefer to face the door without being too close to it, so they do not feel startled if someone enters. Avoid placing the bed right against a window if outside noises or light are an issue.

Lesser-Known Tip: Some believe that having the head of the bed against a solid wall can create a sense of stability. This is not a strict rule, but it might help some people feel less exposed.

---

6. Bedding and Fabrics

Sheets and Blankets

Your bedding can impact how comfortable you feel. Cotton is breathable, while flannel is cozy in colder months. Synthetics might cause sweating for some people, though new fabrics can be both soft and cool. Layering blankets lets you adjust your warmth during the night.

Wash Frequency

Washing sheets often can reduce dust, sweat buildup, and allergens. Some people sleep better with fresh bedding because it has a clean, gentle smell. In warm climates or for those who sweat at night, washing sheets once a week is helpful.

Lesser-Known Tip: Some find that using a weighted blanket can help them relax. The gentle pressure might reduce tossing and turning for certain individuals.

---

7. Scents and Smells

Some smells can keep you awake, like strong cooking odors or intense chemicals. Other smells may help you wind down. A mild aroma from certain gentle oils can signal to the brain that it is time to calm down. Be careful not to use strong fragrances that could irritate allergies or cause headaches.

Lesser-Known Tip: Placing a small dish of plain baking soda under the bed can help absorb unwanted smells in a stuffy room.

---

8. Cleanliness and Clutter

Mental Effect of a Cluttered Room

A messy bedroom can create mild stress. You might see piles of clothes or random objects and feel reminded of chores. This can make it harder to mentally switch off at night. Keeping the room tidy can help you feel relaxed.

Storage

Consider getting drawers or bins that fit under the bed or in the closet for items that otherwise would be scattered around. When things have a set place, it is easier to keep the space neat.

Lesser-Known Tip: Some people find that making the bed each morning adds a small feeling of order and can set the tone for the entire day.

---

9. Electronics in the Bedroom

We will focus more on technology in the next chapter, but for now, remember that televisions, computers, and gaming systems can make it harder to turn off mentally. The light and noise they generate can disrupt rest. Whenever possible, keep your bedroom as a space for rest, not a second entertainment room. If you need a phone alarm, consider putting the phone face-down or using a night mode that keeps the screen dim.

---

10. Bedroom Colors

Soothing Tones

Bright or neon colors can be stimulating. Soft shades like light blues, grays, greens, or neutrals are often considered relaxing to the eyes. That does not mean you must paint your room a dull color, but be aware that very intense shades might keep the mind alert.

Accent Items

If you do want pops of bright color, consider adding them in small items like cushions or artwork rather than on large walls. This way, you still have some energy in the decor without overwhelming the main sleeping area.

Lesser-Known Tip: Matte paint finishes can absorb more light than glossy ones, leading to a calmer look.

11. Plants in the Room

A few indoor plants can help clean the air and add a peaceful touch. Some low-maintenance options might include certain varieties known for filtering common pollutants. Be sure to pick plants that do not produce strong pollen or scents. Also, ensure they are not moldy or overwatered, as that can harm air quality.

Lesser-Known Tip: Certain plant types might produce oxygen at night rather than in the day. Some folks believe this can slightly improve air freshness in the room, though the effect might be modest.

12. Pets and Sleep

Many people love having pets nearby, but pets can disturb sleep. A dog might move around or bark at night, while a cat might knock things over or try to wake you for food. Some people sleep best when pets are not allowed on the bed or sometimes not even in the bedroom. Others find comfort in having them close. It is a personal choice.

Lesser-Known Tip: If you do allow pets in the bedroom, place a separate pet bed in a corner. This can give them a cozy spot and reduce them waking you if they move around.

13. Smart Storage of Distracting Items

If you have work documents, exercise gear, or other reminders of tasks, store them out of sight before bedtime. The bedroom should signal rest, not tasks to be done. If you must keep a desk in your room, keep it tidy at night or use a cover or curtain to block it visually.

Lesser-Known Tip: A simple folding screen can hide an area that is not visually restful, such as a desk or shelving unit loaded with items. This helps the room look calmer when you are ready to sleep.

---

14. Seasonal Adjustments

Your sleep environment may need to change with the seasons:

- **Winter**: Layer the bed with blankets or flannel sheets. A small space heater can help if it is very cold, but make sure it is safe and not left unattended.
- **Summer**: Use lighter sheets, turn on fans, or open windows if the night air is cool. If you have air conditioning, do not set it too cold, as that can also disrupt rest.
- **Allergy Season**: If you are prone to allergies, consider extra dusting, washing bedding more often, and possibly using an air purifier.

Lesser-Known Tip: Switching to different bedding sets each season can also make your room feel fresh. This change can be a small mental cue that suits the changing temperature.

---

15. Personal Touches vs. Overstimulation

It is good to add personal touches, such as photos or decorations that make you feel happy and safe. However, too many visually busy items can overstimulate the brain, especially if they are bright or cluttered. A moderate amount of simple decor can create a balanced environment.

Lesser-Known Tip: Try placing a few calming images or artwork at eye level. Photos of natural scenes or simple abstract designs can soothe the mind without drawing too much attention.

---

16. Gadgets for Comfort

White Noise Devices

We mentioned white noise briefly, but you can also get gadgets that produce other steady sounds like ocean waves, rain, or gentle wind. These can help mask sudden noises from outside.

Air Purifiers

If you live in an area with air pollution or lots of dust, an air purifier can help keep the room fresh. Make sure to clean or replace filters as recommended.

Aromatherapy Diffusers

Some people find diffusers useful, but choose mild scents and run them only for a short time if you are sensitive. Be careful with open flames or heated devices. Safety comes first.

---

17. Safety and Peace of Mind

Feeling safe helps you relax. Check the locks on windows and doors so that you do not worry about intruders. Keep pathways clear of clutter so you can walk around safely at night if you need the bathroom. If you have items that cause you to worry, like important documents or valuables, keep them in a locked drawer or another room, so they are not on your mind.

Lesser-Known Tip: Some people feel calmer when they have a small nightlight in the hallway so that if they wake up, they can see enough to move around without worry. Choose a low-watt bulb or a red-toned light so it does not disrupt rest.

18. Room Arrangement and Mood

The feeling of your space can affect how quickly you wind down:

- **Space Between Furniture**: Having too many things crammed in can create a sense of chaos. Consider rearranging so you can move around easily.
- **Neat Surfaces**: A bedside table filled with random items can be distracting. Keep only what you need at night, like a lamp, a book, or a water glass.
- **Flooring**: If you have a loud or cold floor surface, consider placing a soft rug near the bed. This can be comforting and reduce echoes.

---

19. Testing and Tweaking

You might not get your sleep environment perfect in one go. Try different settings:

- Adjust the room temperature up or down a few degrees.
- Experiment with different pillow heights.
- Place a fan in a new spot to see if the airflow feels better.
- Try room-darkening curtains vs. blinds.

Track any changes in a small notebook or on your phone. See if you notice improvements in how quickly you fall asleep or how often you wake up.

Lesser-Known Tip: If you have a partner, work together on changes, since both of you need to feel at ease. You may need small compromises, like an extra blanket for one person who feels cold while the other prefers the room cool.

---

20. Putting It All Together

A well-organized, tidy, and calm room can support better rest. Factors like temperature, light, noise, and the layout of furniture can either help you feel at ease or keep you awake. Focus on small steps: keep the room clean, make sure the bed is comfy, lower lights before bed, and keep electronic distractions away.

Over time, these changes can make a huge difference in how quickly you fall asleep and how deeply you rest.

Key Points to Remember:

1. **Temperature**: Aim for cool but not freezing.
2. **Darkness**: Use blackout curtains or a mask if needed.
3. **Noise**: Try earplugs, white noise, or heavy curtains to reduce sounds.
4. **Cleanliness**: A tidy space helps calm the mind.
5. **Bedding**: Choose materials that feel comfortable and supportive.
6. **Small Personal Touches**: A few items that bring peace are good, but avoid clutter.

By taking time to shape the bedroom into a calm zone, you give yourself a better chance of experiencing restful nights. In the next chapter, we will address how technology affects rest. We will look at common mistakes people make by using devices late into the evening and discuss ways to use technology wisely if you do not want to give it up entirely.

Chapter 6: Impact of Technology on Sleep

Technology has become a huge part of daily life. Phones, tablets, laptops, and other devices keep us connected around the clock. While these tools can be helpful, they can also interfere with your rest if used in certain ways or at certain times. In this chapter, we will look at how technology can disrupt sleep and explore some tips for handling devices so that they do not ruin your nights.

1. Why Tech Disrupts Rest

Blue Light

Electronic screens emit light in a range of wavelengths, including blue. Blue light can trick the brain into thinking it is still daytime, lowering the body's natural signals to wind down. Usually, the body produces specific hormones in the evening, letting you know it is time to sleep. When you stare at a bright screen, this release can be delayed or reduced.

Mental Stimulation

Even if you use a brightness filter, playing games, reading intense headlines, or engaging in social media can keep your mind active. When you finally put the device away, your thoughts may still be racing. This can make it harder to drift into deeper stages of rest.

Constant Alerts

Notifications, buzzing, and blinking lights can wake you up or at least nudge you into lighter sleep stages. If your phone is nearby, you may check it without thinking, leading to more disruption.

2. Common Bedtime Tech Habits

Scrolling Social Media

Many people habitually scroll through feeds right before turning off the light. Posts might trigger emotional reactions, like excitement or worry, which do not help you calm down. You could stumble on bad news or find yourself comparing your life to someone else's highlights.

Binge-Watching Shows

Watching multiple episodes of a show late at night can cause you to lose track of time. Before you know it, you have stayed up an hour or two past your usual bedtime. The show itself might be thrilling, raising your adrenaline and making rest more difficult.

Gaming

Interactive games can be even more stimulating than watching shows. Fast action can raise your heart rate, and the excitement can stay in your mind. Also, online gaming involves chatting with other players, which can extend the active period of your mind well into the late hours.

---

3. How Phones Affect Sleep Cycles

Phones are especially tricky because they are small, portable, and always close by. If you use your phone in bed, you are training your brain to associate the bed with activity rather than rest. Instead of relaxing as soon as you lie down, your brain might expect to see messages or videos. This can disrupt the natural shift into deeper sleep stages.

Lesser-Known Tip: Some phone activities, such as intense news reading, can cause spikes in stress hormones. These spikes can take hours to return to normal, even if the screen is not as bright as a computer.

4. Specific Device Features That Keep You Awake

Brightness Settings

Most devices let you adjust brightness. A screen set to maximum brightness in a dark room is like shining a flashlight in your eyes. Even if you lower it, if you hold the device close to your face, the effect remains strong.

Color Temperature

Many phones and tablets have a "night mode" that shifts the color temperature of the display, reducing blue light. While this can help, it is not a magic fix. The content you view can still excite your mind.

Vibrations and Sounds

Even if you put your device on silent, small vibrations from notifications can keep you half-alert. The result is more awakenings or partial arousals during the night.

---

5. Handling Social Media and Messaging

Setting Limits

If you find yourself scrolling for hours, consider time limits. Many phones have features that let you set daily app usage caps. You can also download productivity apps that block social media for certain periods.

Evening "Offline" Zones

Try picking a time—maybe 1 or 2 hours before bed—when you stop checking messages or social feeds. Let friends and family know you will be offline. Some people worry they will miss something important, but often the benefits of better sleep are worth the small risk of delayed responses.

Group Chats

Group chats can be active at all hours. You may silence notifications or use "do not disturb" settings. If something urgent happens, people can call you directly, which you might keep as an exception on your phone.

6. Streaming Services

Shows and videos can be a big draw late at night. The auto-play feature on some platforms queues the next episode automatically, so you might end up watching more than planned. Disabling auto-play can give you a clear stop point, reminding you to close the app or turn off the device.

Lesser-Known Tip: Some streaming services allow you to remove certain content from your suggestions. If you know you are likely to keep watching a particularly gripping show, consider hiding it or removing it from your watch list until you have more free time earlier in the day.

7. Video Games

Gaming requires hand-eye coordination and quick thinking. This can be fun, but it can also make your heart rate go up. If you are playing online with friends, you might chat about game tactics, adding more mental energy. When you turn the game off, your mind may stay in "gaming mode" for a while.

Strategies:

- Shift gaming sessions to late afternoon or early evening.
- Choose calmer games if you must play closer to bedtime.
- Take breaks to let your heart rate settle before lying down.

8. E-Readers

E-readers can be a good choice if they have e-ink displays that do not emit the same kind of light as phones or tablets. However, if you have a backlit e-reader or you read on a tablet, that light can still disrupt your sleep.

Workaround: Try a dim reading lamp and a physical book. This reduces screen exposure and can be more relaxing. If you do not want physical books, choose an e-ink reader or lower the brightness if it is backlit.

9. "Smart" Home Devices

Voice assistants and smart speakers can be helpful, but they might also make random noises or light up if they detect motion or hear a sound. Some people have been startled in the middle of the night by an unexpected voice or beep.

Suggestion:

- Turn off non-essential notifications or random "assistant features" at night.
- Place the device away from the bed so any lights or sounds are not disruptive.

---

10. How Late-Night Emails Affect Mental State

Work emails received at night can trigger worry. You might see a task request or a problem that needs solving in the morning, and this can keep your mind active. If you constantly check your inbox, you might never truly relax.

Ideas:

- Only check emails once in the early evening, then log out.
- Let colleagues know you will address late emails the next morning if they are not urgent.
- If you worry about missing something important, you can set a special alert for emails from certain people, like your boss.

---

11. Overthinking Online Content

Reading certain posts, news stories, or online discussions can trigger worry or frustration. These emotions release stress hormones that stay in your system. If you do this close to bedtime, you are basically telling your body to stay alert.

Tip: Seek out lighter or neutral content in the evening, if you must go online. Or pick up a calming physical book or do a simple puzzle. The mind will be more likely to settle that way.

12. Physical Effects of Holding Devices

Hunching over a phone or laptop can strain your neck and shoulders, causing muscle tension. This tension can linger when you try to sleep, especially if you do not stretch or shift position. Some get headaches or eye strain from too much screen time.

Help:

- Take short breaks from screens if you have to use them at night.
- Do a few shoulder rolls or neck stretches before bed to reduce tension.
- Keep devices at eye level when possible, so you are not bending your neck.

---

13. Technology's Role in Our Internal Clock

Your body has a clock that regulates when you feel awake and when you feel sleepy. Bright light at night can push this clock back, leading you to feel more awake than normal in the late hours. Over time, this might cause a delayed sleep schedule.

Lesser-Known Tip: Even if you have the screen brightness low, certain devices still produce enough light to signal the brain that it is not fully dark. This is why experts often say it is best to stop screen usage at least 30 minutes (ideally 60 to 120 minutes) before bedtime.

---

14. Tech to Help You Sleep Better

Not all technology is bad for rest. Some devices or apps can assist your nighttime routine:

- **Calming Sound Apps**: These can generate white noise, nature sounds, or gentle music.
- **Meditation Apps**: Guided sessions can help you relax. Just make sure the screen is dim and you are not also getting notifications.

- **Sleep Tracking Gadgets**: Wearables that track movement and heart rate can offer insights, though they are not always perfect.

Note: Use these tools with caution. Obsessing over nightly stats can cause more worry, which might harm rest. The main goal is to learn patterns and then make healthy changes.

---

15. Setting Tech Boundaries

If you share a home with others, talk about tech rules in shared spaces. For instance, you might agree that after a certain time, the TV goes off or becomes limited to calm shows. For your personal bedroom, consider these boundaries:

- Keep charging stations in another room.
- Use a regular alarm clock instead of a phone alarm.
- Turn off Wi-Fi on devices that do not need updates at night.

---

16. Handling Late-Night Work Emergencies

Some jobs require you to be on call. If you must stay available, consider setting a specific ringtone or text tone for urgent calls. That way, you can silence other notifications but still wake up if something truly important happens. This is better than keeping all alerts active, which can lead to frequent disruptions.

Lesser-Known Tip: Some phones let you set "favorites" or "priority contacts." Only those individuals can bypass silent mode. This can help if you do not want every app or random number waking you up.

---

17. Effects of Watching Bright Screens in the Dark

Watching a screen in a pitch-black room increases the difference between the bright screen and your surroundings. This can strain the eyes and affect sleep signals more strongly. If you must use a screen, keep a soft lamp on so the contrast is less severe, or lower the screen brightness as much as possible.

18. Late-Night Online Shopping

Shopping apps and websites are often designed to grab attention with big images or sales. Browsing these late at night can be more stimulating than you expect. You might buy impulsively or keep scrolling deals, losing track of time.

Strategy: Set a rule that all non-essential shopping ends by a certain hour. If you find something interesting, bookmark it to review the next day. This prevents late-night spending and gives you time to think about whether you really need it.

19. Preparing Devices for Bedtime

Just as you might follow a bedtime routine for yourself, do so for your devices:

1. **Turn Off Unneeded Notifications**: This includes email, social media, and app updates.
2. **Enable "Night Light" or "Night Mode"**: If you really must read something, this reduces some of the harsh light.
3. **Set a Charging Spot**: Put your device in that spot each night so it is not right next to you in bed.

Lesser-Known Tip: Some devices have a "reading mode" that is greyscale. This can reduce some of the excitement that comes from bright app icons and images, helping you stay calmer if you need the device for a brief task.

20. Final Thoughts on Technology and Sleep

Technology can be both a friend and a foe for restful nights. While screens can stimulate the mind and disrupt the body's signals, a few tweaks can lessen the impact. Creating boundaries, using calming tools instead of stimulating content, and giving yourself at least some screen-free time before bed are simple but powerful steps. You do not have to abandon your devices altogether, but you do need to handle them wisely if better rest is your goal.

Key Points to Remember:

1. **Blue Light Delays Sleep**: Use night mode or turn devices off at least an hour before bedtime.
2. **Notifications Are Distracting**: Silence or limit them, especially group chats or social media alerts.
3. **Mind Stimulation**: Content that raises your emotions can keep you awake, so pick calmer activities at night.
4. **Set Boundaries**: Decide on tech-free zones or times in your home.
5. **Use Helpful Apps**: Calming sound apps or gentle meditation guides can support rest if used thoughtfully.

By taking control of how and when you use screens, you can protect your evenings and nights. This ensures that modern tools serve you, rather than robbing you of precious rest. In the next chapters, we will look at nutrition, exercise, and other daytime habits that can affect how soundly you sleep. Each piece of the puzzle is important, and learning to manage technology is a major step toward better sleep.

Chapter 7: Nutrition and Sleep

What we eat affects our entire body, including how well we rest. Many people know that having a large meal right before bed can upset the stomach and make it tough to fall asleep. But nutrition and sleep have more layers than that. In this chapter, we will look at how food choices, mealtimes, and certain nutrients can affect the way we rest. We will also share less-common tips, so you can adjust your diet in ways that support better sleep without feeling like you have to follow a complex plan.

1. Why Food and Sleep Are Linked

Our bodies use nutrients from food to build and repair tissues, create hormones, and produce energy. The sleep-wake cycle depends partly on these processes. When nutrient levels in the body are steady, we can relax more easily. When they swing up and down, we might experience restlessness or nighttime awakenings.

Blood Sugar Balance

After you eat, your blood sugar rises. The body responds by releasing certain hormones that manage how sugar is used or stored. Large spikes and drops in blood sugar can trigger energy surges or crashes, which might show up at night as restlessness or sudden awakenings. Keeping blood sugar more stable through balanced meals can help you rest well.

2. The Timing of Meals

Big Meals at Night

Many people enjoy a hearty dinner, but eating a large, heavy meal right before bed can cause problems. The body needs time to digest. If you lie down immediately, you might experience reflux or heartburn, which can lead to waking up several times. A bloated feeling can also disrupt the body's comfort level, making it tough to settle into deeper sleep stages.

Suggestion: Aim to have your main meal at least two to three hours before bed. This gives the digestive system some time to work through the bulk of the meal. If you are still hungry closer to bedtime, pick a light snack rather than a second big meal.

Skipping Meals

On the other hand, going to bed very hungry can also hurt rest. The body might send signals that it needs fuel, causing you to wake up early or sleep lightly. Striking a balance is key. If dinner is very early and you do not plan to sleep until late, a light snack can keep hunger away.

Less-Known Tip: If you find yourself waking up too early, it could be that your blood sugar is dropping in the early morning hours. A small, balanced snack in the evening—such as a piece of fruit with a bit of protein—might help.

Late-Night Snacks

A light snack before bed can be useful, but picking the right food is important. Protein and complex carbs are more stabilizing than sugary treats. For instance, having a piece of whole-grain toast with peanut butter may be better than sugary cereal or a cookie. The toast-peanut butter combo offers protein, healthy fats, and slower-digesting carbs.

---

3. Specific Nutrients That Affect Rest

Protein and Amino Acids

Protein contains amino acids that help form the body's tissues and make important chemicals in the brain. One amino acid, called tryptophan, is known to help produce certain hormones involved in rest. Some people have heard that turkey has a lot of tryptophan, which can make you feel a bit sleepy after a holiday meal, but turkey is not the only source. Other good sources include beans, nuts, seeds, and some dairy products.

Less-Known Tip: While tryptophan can help, it often works best when eaten along with some carbohydrates. Carbs can help the body move tryptophan into the brain more easily. That is why a balanced meal matters more than focusing on just one amino acid.

Carbohydrates

Carbohydrates are the body's main source of quick energy. Simple carbs (like those in candy or pastries) can cause sharp blood sugar rises and drops, which might lead to poor sleep if eaten too close to bedtime. Complex carbs (found in whole grains, vegetables, and legumes) break down more slowly, maintaining a steadier energy level.

Fats

Healthy fats, such as those in avocados, nuts, seeds, and certain fish, support many body functions. They can also help with feeling satisfied after a meal. On the other hand, eating heavy, greasy foods before bed can lead to digestive upset. Balance is key here, too.

Micronutrients

Vitamins and minerals, though needed in smaller amounts, play a big part in sleep. For example:

1. **Magnesium**: Helps relax muscles and calm the nervous system. Low magnesium might lead to restless nights. Foods like spinach, almonds, and pumpkin seeds are good sources.
2. **Calcium**: Plays a role in producing hormones linked to rest. Dairy products, fortified plant milks, and leafy greens can help meet needs.
3. **Zinc**: Important for overall health, including immune function, which can indirectly affect how well you rest.
4. **B Vitamins**: These help form energy and support nervous system function. Some help in hormone production as well.

Less-Known Tip: Low levels of magnesium, in particular, are often overlooked. If you have frequent muscle cramps or twitchy legs at night, it might be worth checking your intake of magnesium-rich foods or talking to a health professional.

4. Caffeine and Other Stimulants

Caffeine is a major factor in many people's daily routine. It is found in coffee, tea, energy drinks, chocolate, and some medications. While caffeine can help with alertness, it can stay in the body for hours. Consuming it too late can hinder your ability to fall asleep.

How Caffeine Affects Sleep

Caffeine blocks certain receptors in the brain that signal tiredness. Even if you can fall asleep after having caffeine, the depth of your rest might be reduced. You might miss out on deeper stages or wake up earlier than planned.

Less-Known Tip: The half-life of caffeine can be around 5 to 6 hours, depending on the individual. That means if you drink a cup of coffee at 4:00 pm, half of that caffeine could still be in your system by 9:00 or 10:00 pm. Some people process caffeine more slowly than others, so keep track of how it affects you.

Decaf and Alternatives

For those who enjoy the taste of coffee or tea, decaf versions can be an option. Keep in mind that decaf coffee and some teas still have a small amount of caffeine, though usually much less. Herbal teas without caffeine (like chamomile or certain mint blends) can be calming.

Caution: Some herbal teas, especially if they are blends that promote alertness or contain certain plants, might still have stimulating effects. Always check labels if you are sensitive to various herbs.

---

5. Alcohol and Sleep

Many people think that a drink or two in the evening helps them relax and drift off. While alcohol can indeed make you feel sleepy at first, it disrupts the latter parts of the night. You are more likely to wake up in the early hours feeling unsettled or thirsty, and your overall rest quality may drop. Alcohol can reduce the time you spend in deeper stages of rest and shift how you progress through your sleep cycles.

Less-Known Tip: Drinking alcohol before bed can also worsen snoring or breathing problems. It relaxes throat muscles, which may heighten the risk of snoring or more serious issues like obstructive sleep apnea.

6. Hidden Sleep Busters in Food

High Sugar Desserts

Some desserts are very high in sugar. Eating them close to bedtime can lead to a sugar surge, followed by a crash in the middle of the night. That can cause you to wake up at odd hours, or just have restless, shallow sleep.

Spicy Foods

Spicy dishes can lead to acid reflux or heartburn if eaten late. While mild spices might not bother everyone, very hot meals might raise body temperature and disrupt the normal cooling process that helps you fall asleep.

Large Amounts of Fluids

Staying hydrated is good, but drinking excessive fluids too close to bedtime can lead to multiple bathroom trips. If you find yourself waking up often, consider limiting fluids in the last hour or two before sleep, focusing on steady intake during the day instead.

7. Special Foods That May Help Rest

Although no single food will act like a magic wand for sleep, certain foods contain nutrients that can support rest.

1. **Kiwi**: Some research suggests that kiwi might support better rest. It has vitamins, minerals, and antioxidants that may help regulate body processes.
2. **Tart Cherries**: Contain small amounts of natural compounds that can aid in hormone balance related to rest. Some people drink tart cherry juice before bed.

3. **Nuts and Seeds**: These provide magnesium, healthy fats, and some protein. Almonds, walnuts, and pumpkin seeds are popular picks.
4. **Oats**: Whole oats are a source of complex carbs and some vitamins. A small bowl of oatmeal with milk can be comforting and filling if you need a light evening snack.

Less-Known Tip: Some individuals mix a small amount of tart cherry juice with water to reduce the sugar content and still get the potential rest-related benefits.

---

8. Emotional Eating and Sleep

Stress can cause people to eat more or less than normal. Emotional eating might lead to consuming high-calorie or sugary foods late at night, which can disrupt rest. On the flip side, some people lose their appetite when anxious and go to bed hungry, which can also cause trouble.

Strategies:

- Take a short pause when you feel the urge to eat late at night. Ask yourself if you are truly hungry or if you are stressed, bored, or upset.
- Keep healthy snack options available, like fruit or yogurt, so that if you do eat late, you are not filling up on junk food.
- If you find yourself eating too little because of stress, plan your meals ahead of time, so you get enough nutrients to keep your body balanced.

---

9. Fasting and Sleep

Some people try various forms of fasting, such as skipping meals or having a strict eating window each day. While fasting can help some individuals with metabolism or other goals, it can also affect rest. If you skip dinner or delay breakfast, your body might produce certain hormones that interfere with normal sleep patterns.

Tips:

- If you are trying a new eating approach like intermittent fasting, observe how it affects your rest over a week or two.
- If you notice an increase in nighttime awakenings or more difficulty falling asleep, consider adjusting your meal times.
- Make sure you get enough nutrients during the eating window, so you are not going to bed with a nutrient deficiency.

---

10. Social and Cultural Factors

In some cultures, dinner is a light meal, while others might have their biggest meal late at night. Patterns like these can be deeply ingrained. If you live in a place where late dinners are common, you can still adapt by choosing lighter dishes or allowing more time after dinner before lying down.

Less-Known Tip: If late-evening dinners are a cultural norm, a small walk or gentle stretching session after the meal can aid digestion. This might help your body wind down more easily once bedtime arrives.

---

11. Supplements and Sleep Aids

Common Supplements

- **Melatonin**: A hormone the body makes naturally, often sold in pill form. Some people use it to help reset their body clock or manage jet lag.
- **Magnesium**: Available in several forms. Some claim it can reduce muscle tension and promote calm feelings before bed.
- **Herbal Mixes**: Various herbal supplements advertise better rest. Always check with a health professional to avoid interactions with medications.

Warning: Taking supplements without understanding your body's needs can lead to imbalances. Too much of any nutrient can cause side effects or interfere with other nutrients. Always do your research or consult an expert if you have concerns.

12. Daytime Eating Habits That Support Nighttime Rest

Balanced Breakfast

Starting the day with a balanced meal can reduce cravings and blood sugar spikes later. This can set the tone for stable energy levels. If you skip breakfast, you might overeat at lunch, which can shift your overall daily food intake toward the evening, increasing the chance of nighttime discomfort.

Consistent Meal Times

A regular eating schedule trains your body to expect fuel at certain points in the day. This can help manage hunger hormones, which in turn support a healthy sleep-wake cycle. If your meal times shift daily, your body might struggle with confusion around energy and rest.

Hydration

Drinking enough water during the day is important. Mild dehydration can lead to headaches, low energy, and trouble focusing, which might cause you to reach for caffeinated drinks that interfere with sleep. By staying properly hydrated from morning to early evening, you can reduce thirst at night and avoid too many bathroom trips.

13. Allergies and Food Sensitivities

Food sensitivities can lead to bloating, inflammation, and discomfort that disturb rest. Common triggers include dairy, wheat, soy, eggs, or certain nuts. If you suspect a sensitivity, keep a food diary and note when you experience rest problems, stomach pains, or skin reactions. Over time, you can see patterns and adjust your diet.

Less-Known Tip: Some people experience delayed reactions to certain foods, meaning the discomfort might not show up until several hours after eating. This can be tricky to connect to sleep problems. A detailed journal can help you spot the link.

14. Foods That Calm the Mind

Some foods might help calm the nervous system. These are not guaranteed cures, but they can be part of a soothing routine:

- **Warm Milk**: Known for its tryptophan content, and the warmth can be comforting.
- **Herbal Teas**: Certain blends labeled as "sleepy" or "nighttime" may contain chamomile, which is often used for calmness.
- **Bananas**: Contain potassium and magnesium, which can help relax muscles.

Note: If you are lactose-intolerant, warm dairy milk might not be a good choice. Try lactose-free milk or a non-dairy option that you tolerate well.

---

15. Less-Common Nutritional Tips for Sleep

1. **Glycine-Rich Foods**: Glycine is an amino acid that may help calm the brain. It is found in foods like bone broth, poultry, and certain cuts of meat. Some prefer to get glycine from supplements, but dietary sources are often good if tolerated.
2. **Limit Strong Aromas**: Powerful flavors like garlic or onions can linger, causing heartburn for some people when eaten too close to bedtime.
3. **Evening Ritual Snacks**: Some individuals stick to the same calming snack each night, like half a banana with a spoonful of nut butter. Over time, the body associates that snack with bedtime, which can help form a mental cue.

---

16. Mindful Eating and Relaxation

Rushing through meals or eating while distracted (watching TV or scrolling on the phone) can lead to overeating or poor digestion. Mindful eating involves paying attention to textures, flavors, and feelings of fullness. When you slow down at dinner, you may experience fewer digestive troubles at bedtime.

Simple Mindful Steps

- Put your fork or spoon down between bites.
- Take a sip of water now and then.
- Notice the taste and smell of each mouthful.
- Stop when you feel satisfied, not stuffed.

17. Stress-Eating Patterns

When stressed, some people reach for sugary or high-fat foods. While these might provide a brief sense of comfort, they can disrupt blood sugar and lead to restless nights. Try to address the source of stress instead of soothing it only with food. Use other calming methods like taking a short walk, doing a breathing exercise, or chatting with a friend.

18. Planning Your Evening Meals

One way to ensure a good nutritional balance at dinner (or your last meal of the day) is to include a mix of protein, healthy fats, and carbs with fiber. Examples:

- **Grilled Fish + Brown Rice + Steamed Vegetables**
- **Tofu Stir-Fry with Vegetables + Whole-Grain Noodles**
- **Chicken or Bean Soup with Whole-Grain Bread**

Such balanced meals can help keep blood sugar steady and reduce the chance of big spikes or crashes.

19. Moderation and Personal Differences

Everyone's body reacts differently. Some people can eat spicy curry an hour before bed and sleep fine. Others might need at least three hours after a meal to rest comfortably. Pay attention to how your body responds. Keep a small log for a few weeks noting:

- What you ate at dinner.
- How you slept that night (time to fall asleep, any awakenings, how you felt in the morning).

You might spot patterns like, "Every time I have extra-spicy food close to bedtime, I wake up at 2 am" or "If I skip a snack, I wake up hungry at 4 am." Once you see a trend, you can make adjustments.

---

20. Conclusion and Next Steps

Eating well is not just about fueling the body for daytime tasks. It also sets the stage for restful nights. By choosing balanced meals, watching your meal timing, and focusing on nutrients that support calmness, you can help your body relax. Avoiding large, sugary, or spicy meals near bedtime can prevent physical discomfort, while mindful eating helps you notice signals from your body. If you handle your nutrition with awareness, you will likely see improvements in how easily you fall asleep and how refreshed you feel in the morning.

Key Points:

1. Big, heavy meals right before bed can cause discomfort.
2. Balanced snacks with protein and complex carbs are better than sugary treats at night.
3. Caffeine and alcohol can disrupt rest if consumed late.
4. Certain nutrients (magnesium, tryptophan) support a calmer mind.
5. Keep track of your habits to see what works best for you.

In the next chapter, we will talk about the importance of physical activity for rest. Many people do not realize how much exercise can help regulate the body's sleep-wake cycle. We will share ways to move more during the day, along with special pointers that are not always well-known, so you can get the most from your workouts without interfering with your nights.

Chapter 8: Importance of Exercise

In the previous chapter, we looked at how nutrition affects rest. Now it is time to discuss another key factor: physical activity. Exercise helps with weight management, heart health, and muscle strength, but it also plays a major part in how well you sleep. When you get the right amount and type of movement, your body is more likely to settle down at night and achieve deeper rest. In this chapter, we will explore many aspects of exercise and how they tie into sleep, along with less-familiar tips you might not have heard elsewhere.

1. How Exercise Helps the Body Rest

Tiring Out the Muscles

One straightforward reason exercise supports rest is that it uses energy. When muscles work, they become tired. By the end of the day, the body often wants to recover, which can lead to better sleep quality.

Balancing Hormones

Physical activity affects hormone levels. It can boost mood-supporting chemicals and help regulate stress hormones. People who work out regularly often have lower resting levels of stress chemicals, making it easier to relax at night.

Improving Blood Flow

Exercise increases circulation, delivering oxygen and nutrients throughout the body. This can help with overall health, which in turn supports better rest. A healthy body generally has an easier time transitioning between sleep stages without frequent awakenings.

2. Different Types of Exercise and Their Effects

Aerobic Activities

These include running, walking, cycling, swimming, or anything that gets your heart rate up for a sustained period. Aerobic workouts often lead to improvements in cardiovascular health, which can support stable rest. However, doing intense aerobics right before bedtime can energize you too much, so it is usually best to finish such workouts a few hours earlier.

Lesser-Known Tip: Some people find moderate evening walks helpful. They are not too intense but can help settle the mind and body.

Strength Training

Lifting weights or doing resistance exercises helps build and maintain muscle. It can also improve metabolism. Strength training can be done at various times of the day. Some people worry that late-night strength workouts will keep them awake. This depends on intensity. A heavy workout might raise your heart rate and temperature for a while, but many find that once their bodies cool down, they sleep deeply.

Stretching and Flexibility

Gentle yoga-like stretches, as well as simple floor exercises, can help loosen tight muscles. This can relieve tension that might keep you from feeling comfortable in bed. Stretching before bedtime should be calm and not too vigorous.

Balance and Functional Movement

Activities that develop coordination—like certain bodyweight routines or low-impact sports—also help you become more aware of your body. Better coordination can reduce stress on joints, making aches less likely to disturb your rest.

---

3. How Much Exercise Do You Need?

There is no single answer for everyone, but health groups often recommend at least 150 minutes of moderate aerobic activity per week, plus some strength work for major muscle groups on at least two days. When it comes to sleep, consistency is more important than pushing yourself hard just once a week. A daily or near-daily moderate routine tends to help the body settle into a steady rhythm.

Too Little Movement

If you barely move all day—maybe due to a desk job or long commutes—the body may not feel physically ready for rest. You could find yourself feeling restless or wide awake at night, even if your mind is tired.

Too Much Movement

Overtraining can also harm rest. If you exercise at high intensity every day without proper recovery, stress hormones might stay elevated. This can lead to trouble dozing off or waking up in the night with sore muscles or a racing heart. Balance is crucial.

---

4. Best Time of Day to Exercise

Morning Workouts

Some people like working out in the morning. It can give an energy boost and help regulate the circadian rhythm, which is the body's internal clock. Morning exercise might help you fall asleep earlier at night because your body has been active throughout the day.

Caution: Very intense morning workouts could lead to an energy crash midday if you do not refuel properly. Also, it may not be realistic for everyone's schedule.

Afternoon Workouts

Early to mid-afternoon can be a good time if you have free periods. This can break up a sedentary day and keep you from feeling too wired at bedtime. If the afternoon slump is a problem, a short workout might increase alertness for the rest of the day, but not so late that it ruins sleep.

Evening Workouts

Working out too close to bedtime can raise body temperature and heart rate, possibly delaying sleep. However, some moderate activities like brisk walking, light yoga, or gentle stretching in the evening may help you relax. It depends on intensity. If your schedule forces you to exercise late, try cooling down properly and ending at least an hour (or more) before bedtime.

5. Exercise and Stress Management

Physical activity is often recommended to reduce stress. Less stress can mean better rest, as we covered in a previous chapter. Exercise can also provide mental clarity. If you have a stressful job or personal challenges, doing something active can serve as a healthy outlet. By the time you are ready for bed, you have an emotional release and might feel calmer.

Lowering Cortisol

Chronic stress leads to high levels of cortisol, a hormone that keeps you alert. Regular activity can help lower baseline cortisol over time. This means your body is less likely to stay on high alert at bedtime.

Less-Known Tip: Slow, rhythmic workouts, such as swimming laps at a leisurely pace, can be especially good for stress relief because they combine steady movement with regulated breathing patterns.

6. Special Activities for Better Sleep

Tai Chi or Qi Gong

These gentle exercises come from certain cultural traditions and involve slow, intentional movements. They can improve balance, relaxation, and body awareness. Many people say these practices help them sleep better, likely because they lower stress and promote focus on the present moment.

Light Evening Yoga

Not all yoga is the same. Vigorous power yoga can be very intense, but many forms are calm and geared toward relaxation. Simple poses that stretch the back, hips, and shoulders can release tension collected during the day.

Less-Known Tip: If you do yoga right before bed, dim the lights and avoid poses that raise your heart rate too much. Focus on gentle forward bends or seated stretches.

Leisurely Nature Walks

Spending time outdoors can help regulate your internal clock, especially if you do it in the morning or late afternoon. Natural light exposure, combined with mild physical activity, can make your body more in sync with day and night.

7. Exercise for Specific Sleep Problems

1. **Insomnia**: Moderate exercise on a routine schedule can help with insomnia over time. It might take weeks of consistent activity before you see a big improvement, but many find that they fall asleep faster and stay asleep longer.
2. **Sleep Apnea**: Being active and managing weight can sometimes reduce apnea symptoms, especially if there is extra tissue around the neck. While exercise does not "cure" apnea, a stronger respiratory system can help.
3. **Restless Legs**: Gentle stretching and moderate exercise can lessen the urge to move the legs at night. Too much intense activity might worsen the feeling, so keep it balanced.
4. **Circadian Rhythm Issues**: Timed exercise—like morning runs or afternoon workouts—can signal the body about when to be awake and when to rest, helping reset the internal clock.

---

8. Strategies for Staying Active During the Day

Micro Workouts

If you have a busy schedule, try doing small bursts of activity throughout the day. For example, do a set of push-ups or squats during breaks, take the stairs instead of the elevator, or walk to do errands. Over time, these short moments add up and help keep the body from being too sedentary.

Active Commuting

If possible, walk or bike to work or school. Even parking farther away from the building can give you a short walk. This might not seem like much, but daily movement helps the body feel more balanced.

Walking Meetings or Breaks

If your workplace allows, propose walking meetings. Instead of sitting in a conference room, walk around the block while discussing business. Or use your break time to walk instead of just sitting in a lounge. This can improve blood flow and might spark fresh ideas.

9. Avoiding Injury and Overtraining

Proper Form

Rushing into new exercises without learning correct form can lead to strains or pains, which might disrupt rest while your body tries to heal. Take time to learn proper techniques, even for basic moves. If needed, ask a trainer or watch reliable instruction videos.

Rest Days

Your muscles need rest days to recover and rebuild. Overtraining can show up as constant fatigue, poor performance, or frequent colds due to a weakened immune system. Proper rest days or active recovery (like gentle stretching or easy walks) can keep your progress steady without burning out.

Less-Known Tip: Some athletes use foam rolling or massage to help muscles recover. Doing this in the evening can ease tension, but be gentle to avoid too much stimulation.

---

10. Balancing Exercise with Other Daily Activities

If you have a job that requires physical labor, you might not need a separate intense workout each day. Instead, you could focus on specific stretches or targeted exercises to correct muscle imbalances. Conversely, if you sit all day at a computer, aim for more frequent breaks to stand, stretch, or walk.

Practical Example: A construction worker might need a gentle yoga session in the evening to soothe tired muscles, while an office worker could benefit more from a brisk 30-minute walk after work to get the blood flowing.

---

11. Impact of Exercise on Sleep Stages

Deep Sleep (Stage N3)

Physical activity can help increase time spent in deep sleep. This is the stage where the body repairs tissues and recharges. If you are physically active during the day, your body has a strong reason to dive more deeply into recovery at night.

REM Sleep

Being active can also help balance your REM sleep. If you are frequently stressed or anxious, you might have an irregular pattern of REM. Exercise can reduce stress, possibly leading to a healthier distribution of REM cycles.

Less-Known Tip: One or two nights of exercise will not magically boost your deep sleep if the rest of your schedule is out of control. Consistency over weeks or months is what delivers the real benefits.

---

12. Outdoor vs. Indoor Activities

Benefits of Outdoor Activities

- **Natural Light**: Helps reset your internal clock.
- **Fresh Air**: Can improve breathing.
- **Changing Scenery**: Might reduce boredom and stress.

Indoor Gym Workouts

- **Controlled Environment**: Good for extreme weather conditions.
- **Equipment Variety**: Allows you to target specific muscles or track your progress.
- **Social Aspect**: Classes or shared spaces can motivate some people.

Note: Either approach can support better rest. Pick what fits your lifestyle and interests.

---

13. Tech Tools for Exercise

You can use apps or wearable gadgets to track steps, heart rate, or other metrics. This can be motivating, but be careful not to obsess over numbers, as it could create stress. Some tools offer guided workout routines or quick exercises you can do at home.

Caution: Using screens late at night to follow a workout might bring back some of the light-related sleep issues. If possible, complete your guided workouts earlier in the evening, or use a device with minimal brightness.

---

14. Older Adults and Exercise

As people age, muscle mass can decrease, and they might experience stiffness or reduced flexibility. Gentle weight-bearing exercises, walking, and low-impact activities can help maintain strength and balance. This often leads to better rest because aches and pains are less troublesome at night.

Less-Known Tip: Water aerobics can be great for older adults because the water supports the body's weight, reducing impact on joints. This can ease physical strain and lead to more restful nights.

---

15. Teens and Young Adults

Younger people might have high energy and be active naturally if they play sports. However, those who spend a lot of time studying or gaming might not get enough movement. Encouraging regular sports, dance, or even short exercise breaks can help them regulate their internal clock, especially if they tend to stay up late and sleep in.

Practical Approach: Setting a consistent schedule that includes an hour of some activity in the afternoon can make a big difference in a teen's ability to sleep well at night.

---

16. Exercise and Mood Disorders

For individuals dealing with low mood or too much worry, physical activity can be a powerful tool. It raises mood-supporting chemicals in the brain and can boost feelings of well-being. Better mood often links to better rest, since sadness or worry can keep the mind active at night.

Less-Known Tip: Even small activities, like going for a 10-minute walk, can have a noticeable effect on mood, which can then improve rest patterns if done regularly.

---

17. Combining Nutrition and Exercise for Optimal Sleep

From the previous chapter, you learned about how balanced meals help keep energy stable. Pairing this with the right amount of exercise can enhance your sleep even more. For instance, a moderate workout followed by a protein- and carb-rich snack can support muscle recovery, reducing aches and pains that might disturb you at night.

- Example: After a moderate workout, a small smoothie with fruits (carbs) and yogurt (protein) could help stabilize blood sugar and start muscle repair.

---

18. Avoiding Late-Night Adrenaline Surges

High-intensity interval training or highly competitive sports right before bed can elevate adrenaline. You might find yourself lying in bed with a pounding heart. If that is your only available time, be sure to include a thorough cooldown, which might include slow walking, deep breathing, and light stretching. This can help bring your heart rate back down.

---

19. Keeping a Simple Workout Log

To see how movement affects your rest, keep a brief log. Note:

- What type of exercise you did.
- The intensity level (light, moderate, vigorous).
- The time you did it.
- How you slept that night (how long to fall asleep, any awakenings, overall feel in the morning).

Over a month or two, patterns might emerge. Maybe you notice that moderate workouts around 5 pm lead to great rest, while doing them at 9 pm leaves you too wired. This allows you to adjust your routine.

---

20. Bringing It All Together

Exercise is a key part of a healthy lifestyle and plays a direct role in how well you rest. It can help burn off extra energy, lower stress, and support the hormones your body needs for a good night's sleep. The trick is to choose activities you enjoy and schedule them wisely. Overdoing it can lead to the opposite effect, keeping you up at night. Balancing cardio, strength, flexibility, and daily movement routines can make a big difference.

Key Points:

1. Regular physical activity helps tire out the body and mind, promoting deeper rest.
2. Timing matters: intense workouts close to bedtime can be too energizing.
3. Consistency is crucial: build a habit of moderate movement most days of the week.
4. Low-impact or gentle activities in the evening can relax the body without causing restlessness.
5. Track how different exercise types affect your rest, then plan your schedule around those observations.

By adding the right amount of movement into your day—whether it is a walk in the park, a bike ride, light weights, or yoga—you support your body's natural rhythms. In the next chapters, we will continue to address other elements that affect rest, such as light exposure, routines, and practical strategies for building a complete plan to improve your nights. The hope is that each piece you learn helps you fine-tune your sleep habits so you can wake up feeling more refreshed and ready for the day.

Chapter 9: Effects of Light

Light plays a major part in our daily life. It not only helps us see but also guides our bodies as they decide when to be awake and when to rest. In this chapter, we will look at how light affects our internal clocks, how artificial and natural lights differ, and how to adjust your exposure to light for better rest. We will also cover less-common ideas about how to handle changes in daylight during different seasons and how indoor lighting choices might influence your nights.

1. Why Light Matters for Rest

Our bodies have an internal clock, sometimes called the circadian rhythm. This clock runs on a cycle of roughly 24 hours. It regulates when we feel alert and when we feel sleepy. Light is one of the most powerful cues for this clock. When bright light hits our eyes, certain signals travel to the brain, telling it that it is daytime. As a result, the brain lowers the release of certain hormones that encourage rest. When evening comes and things grow dark, the brain increases these hormones, helping the body wind down.

If you receive a lot of bright light at night, it can confuse the clock. The body might think it is still daytime, leading you to feel more awake than you want to be at bedtime. Likewise, if you stay in dim areas during the morning or day, your body may not fully switch into "awake mode," causing grogginess or trouble focusing.

2. Natural Light and the Circadian Rhythm

Natural sunlight is typically brighter than indoor lights. Even a cloudy day can supply a level of brightness far above that of most indoor bulbs. When you step outside in the morning, sunlight enters your eyes, sending a message to the brain that it is time to start the day. This helps set the schedule for hormone release, body temperature changes, and other internal functions.

Less-Known Tip: Spending just 10 to 15 minutes in early morning sunlight can help anchor your internal clock. This small action can help you fall asleep more easily at night because your body knows when the "day" officially started.

Morning Sun vs. Afternoon Sun

Morning sunlight has a special effect on your body's clock. The angle of the sun's rays and the brightness level in the early part of the day appear to be ideal for signaling that it is daytime. If you cannot get morning sun, even stepping outside later in the day for some bright light can still help, but morning exposure is often the most effective.

---

3. Artificial Light and Its Influence

Indoor Lighting

Most homes and offices use artificial lights that might not match the brightness or the color mix of natural daylight. These lights allow us to see at night, but they can also trick the body into staying more alert. Traditional light bulbs emit warm or cool glows, but many do not have the same intensity as sunlight. Some modern LED or fluorescent lights can be quite bright, almost imitating daylight, which can be good for productivity during work hours but can disrupt rest if used late.

Electronic Screens

Phones, tablets, computers, and TVs all emit light. A large part of that light is in the "blue" range of the spectrum. Blue light is especially powerful in telling the brain to stay awake. That is why using screens at night can make it hard to doze off. Even small screens, held close to the face, can shine enough brightness to delay the release of rest-supporting chemicals.

Key Point: If you often scroll in bed, the blue light from your phone can signal the brain that it is still daytime. This means your body might not start the rest process as early as it needs to, delaying deep rest and reducing sleep quality.

4. Blue Light and Sleep Problems

Blue light is not always bad. Sunlight in the morning has plenty of blue waves that help us wake up. The problem is getting blue light too late in the evening. When it is dark outside but your screens or overhead lights are bright, your body's clock receives mixed signals.

Less-Known Tip: Some modern devices come with "night modes" or "blue light filters," which shift the color of the screen to warmer tones. While these can reduce some of the alerting effects, the content on the screen (like exciting shows or intense social media) can still keep your brain active. It is not just the color of the light but also the mental stimulation from the device.

5. Seasonal Changes

In some parts of the world, daylight hours change noticeably with the seasons. During winter, days are shorter, and nights are longer. This can lead to a shift in mood and rest patterns for some people, often called seasonal blues. On the other hand, summertime can bring very long days, making it harder to wind down if the sun stays up late.

Ways to Handle Seasonal Light Changes

- **Use Light Therapy Boxes**: Some people use specially designed lamps that emit bright light, often in the morning, to mimic the effect of natural sunlight.
- **Adjust Your Evening Routine**: If it stays bright until late, consider adding heavier curtains or blinds to darken your home earlier in the evening, so your body can start to relax.
- **Plan Outdoor Time**: In winter, take advantage of any daylight you have. Even a short midday walk can help your body realize it is day, making the early sunset less disruptive.

6. Bright Light in the Evening

If you keep all your lights on, watch bright TV screens, or work under intense lighting at night, your body might not begin releasing rest-promoting hormones at the right time. Think about how, before modern lighting, people relied on candles or oil lamps after sunset. Those are much dimmer and have a warmer hue, which does not disrupt the body's signals as much.

Practical Tip: Start dimming lights about an hour before bedtime. Switch off overhead lights and use small lamps or night lights instead. This gradual shift from bright to dim can help the brain realize that sleep time is near.

---

7. The Role of Color Temperature

Light sources have different "color temperatures," which can range from warm (yellowish) to cool (bluish). Daylight is often considered cool in the middle of the day, but it changes throughout the day's cycle. Many indoor bulbs are labeled as "warm white" or "daylight" bulbs. Warm white bulbs usually have a softer, more yellow tone, which is gentler on the eyes at night.

Less-Known Tip: Some newer smart bulbs let you adjust color temperature. You can set them to a cooler color early in the day (to help you wake up) and switch them to a warm, dim tone in the evening. That helps mimic natural changes in daylight.

---

8. Nighttime Darkness and Blackout Curtains

Total darkness can be a big help for some people. Street lamps, headlights, or brightly lit neighborhoods might shine light into your room all night long. This light can stop you from reaching deeper levels of rest, even if you do not fully wake up. Blackout curtains or blinds can block a lot of that light.

Less-Known Tip: If blackout curtains are not an option (for instance, if you rent a place where you cannot install them), consider using a sleep mask to cover your eyes. A well-fitted mask can create darkness for your eyes, even if the room is not fully dark.

9. Impact of Artificial Night Lights

Some people like to sleep with a small lamp or night light. This can be helpful if you often get up to use the bathroom or if you feel uneasy in total darkness. However, too bright of a night light can still disrupt rest. Look for a dim red or orange night light rather than a bright white or blue one. Red or orange lights are less likely to signal the brain to stay awake.

---

10. Sunrise Alarm Clocks

A sunrise alarm clock is a device that gradually brightens before your set wake-up time, aiming to mimic a natural dawn. The idea is that slow, gentle light can ease you out of rest, making it more pleasant than a sudden beep. This can help your body align with a more natural wake-up rhythm, especially if you need to get up before the sun rises.

Less-Known Tip: Some sunrise clocks also offer sunset features, where the light slowly dims in the evening. This can help calm your mind and signal that it is time to go to bed, mimicking the natural shift from day to night.

---

11. Indoor Work and Lack of Sunlight

A challenge for many is spending the entire day inside. Offices, labs, and even some home settings might have limited windows or rely on weak lighting. If you go all day with dim lighting, your body may not get a strong "daytime" signal. This can lead to feeling tired or unfocused, making you reach for caffeine late in the day, which might then harm your rest.

Practical Ideas

- **Breaks Outside**: Step outdoors briefly, even if only for a few minutes, to get some direct light.
- **Desk Near a Window**: If possible, place your workspace near natural light.
- **Use a Bright Lamp**: If windows are not an option, try a high-lumen daylight lamp during the daytime hours to mimic stronger light.

12. City Lights and Light Pollution

In large cities, light pollution from street lamps, billboards, and buildings can keep the sky from getting truly dark at night. This glow can trickle into bedrooms. Even if it seems dim, it might be enough to keep you from resting as deeply as you could in total darkness.

Solutions

- **Heavier Window Treatments**: Thick curtains or blinds can reduce city glow.
- **Shield Lights**: In some cases, installing or adjusting outdoor fixtures to direct light downward (if it is your property) can help.
- **Rearranging Furniture**: Placing the bed in a spot that gets the least amount of outside light can also be beneficial.

---

13. Light for Shift Workers

If you work nights or rotate between day and night shifts, controlling light exposure becomes more complicated. You might need to mimic nighttime during the day so you can rest after a night shift.

Tips for Shift Workers

- **Wear Dark Sunglasses on the Way Home**: This limits bright morning light that might trick your body into feeling too awake when you should be heading to bed.
- **Use Blackout Curtains**: Make your bedroom as dark as possible, even during daylight hours.
- **Create a Fake Dawn**: When it is time to get up, use bright lights or a sunrise clock to help your brain understand it is "morning," even if real sunlight is out of sync with your schedule.

---

14. Balancing Screen Time with Light Needs

We live in a world where many tasks involve screens. If you must use a computer or phone at night, try these steps:

1. **Screen Filters**: Some free apps and built-in settings can shift the screen color to warmer tones.
2. **Reduce Brightness**: Lower the screen brightness to the lowest comfortable level.
3. **Take Screen Breaks**: Look away from the screen every 15 to 20 minutes. This can lessen eye strain.
4. **Set a Cutoff Time**: Ideally, stop using screens an hour or so before bed.

---

15. Measuring Brightness in Your Room

You can find light meter apps or use handheld tools to measure how bright your room is at different times. This can be helpful if you suspect your environment is too bright or too dim. For bedtime, you want the reading to be very low—close to complete darkness, if possible. During daytime hours, aim for something closer to outdoor levels (or as high as you can manage) to keep your body clock in tune.

Less-Known Tip: You do not have to become obsessed with exact numbers. Just a general sense of whether your space is bright enough in the day and dark enough at night can guide your adjustments.

---

16. The Psychological Aspect of Light

Some folks find that bright light in the evening makes them feel more upbeat, so they might resist dimming the lights. But if the goal is better rest, you can shift your brighter, more active tasks to earlier hours and ease into dimmer light later on. Over time, the mind can adapt to seeing lower light levels in the evening as a sign of relaxation.

---

17. Handling Nighttime Waking with Light

If you must get up during the night—for example, to use the bathroom—try to keep the lights off or very dim. Switching on a bright overhead bulb can jolt your system into thinking it is morning. A small, warm-colored night light can guide your path without waking you too much.

Less-Known Tip: If you are prone to bumping into furniture, place low-level lights with motion sensors near the floor. They will give enough glow for safety but not enough to disrupt your rest hormones.

---

18. Stargazing and Natural Darkness

In rural areas with low light pollution, people sometimes find it easier to rest well because nights are truly dark. Also, stargazing can be a relaxing activity that gets you outside in natural darkness. Even if you cannot see many stars due to city lights, the act of stepping outside and turning off indoor lights for a little while can help your mind calm down and recognize that nighttime has arrived.

---

19. Special Concerns for Children

Children often want night lights because they feel safer. A very dim, warm-colored light is usually best if they need one. For teenagers, late-night device use can be a major source of poor rest. Encouraging healthy phone habits (like no screens in bed) can significantly improve their rest quality.

Practical Idea: Some parents gradually lower the brightness of lights as bedtime approaches, helping children's bodies and minds shift toward a calmer state. This approach can also be used for adults who want a more natural evening wind-down.

---

20. Putting It All Together

Light has a direct and powerful effect on when you feel awake and when you feel ready to rest. By controlling the type, amount, and timing of light exposure, you can help your body maintain a stable schedule. Try these simple actions:

1. **Get Morning Sun**: Step outside soon after waking, or sit by a bright window.
2. **Dim Lights at Night**: Lower overhead lights, use warm lamps, and switch off strong bulbs.
3. **Mind Your Screens**: Use blue light filters or reduce screen use in the last hour before bed.
4. **Block External Light**: Use blackout curtains, blinds, or a sleep mask if outside lights invade your room.
5. **Consider a Sunrise Clock**: Gradual light can be nicer for morning wake-ups.

By making thoughtful changes, you can guide your internal clock back to its natural rhythm. This, in turn, can reduce bedtime tossing and turning, lower nighttime awakenings, and help you wake up feeling more refreshed. In the next chapter, we will explore the role of routine. A regular daily plan can further reinforce the benefits of proper light exposure, nutrition, and activity, helping you achieve consistent, healthy rest.

Chapter 10: The Role of Routine

We have talked about many factors that affect rest, such as stress, the bedroom environment, and exposure to light. In this chapter, we focus on the power of having a routine—both at bedtime and throughout the day. A routine can create predictable signals for the body and mind, making it much easier to drift off at night. We will explore different pieces of a routine, ways to handle unexpected events, and tips to avoid boredom while still maintaining a stable schedule.

1. Why Routine Is Helpful

The human body thrives on regularity. We have hormones that rise and fall in a pattern. When we go to bed and wake up at the same times each day, our internal clock becomes more stable. This stability leads to feeling sleepy at a consistent bedtime and more awake when it is time to start the day. If you change your schedule drastically from one day to the next—staying up late some nights and sleeping early on others—you can confuse that clock, leading to restless nights and drowsy mornings.

Routine vs. Rigidity

Some worry that sticking to a routine will feel too strict. But a routine does not have to be rigid. It can be flexible while still giving enough structure that the body knows what to expect. For example, you can aim for a consistent bedtime within a 30-minute window, rather than an exact minute of the clock.

2. Building a Simple Bedtime Routine

A bedtime routine consists of the actions you take in the hour or two before lights out. These actions serve as cues that tell your brain it is nearly time for rest. It is important to keep it relatively consistent day after day so that your mind and body learn these signals.

Possible elements of a bedtime routine might include:

1. **Dimming Lights**: Start turning off main overhead lights, switching to lamps or low-level bulbs.
2. **Screen Curfew**: Stop using devices or apply night-mode filters.
3. **Personal Hygiene**: A warm shower, gentle face wash, or brushing your teeth.
4. **Relaxing Activity**: Reading a calming book, listening to soothing music, or doing a simple craft.
5. **Mind Practice**: Breathing exercises, writing in a journal, or other calming mental tasks.

---

3. The Timing of Your Bedtime

Picking a bedtime that suits your lifestyle is key. If you have to wake up for work or school at 6:00 am, going to bed at midnight might not allow enough rest. You might aim for 10:00 pm or 10:30 pm, leaving at least seven to eight hours of rest opportunity. If you are someone who naturally feels alert at night, you might need to shift your routine slowly, moving bedtime earlier or later in small steps.

Less-Known Tip: Changing bedtime too fast—like trying to move it two hours earlier all at once—can backfire. A gentler approach is shifting it by 15 minutes each night until you reach the desired schedule. This gives your body time to adapt.

---

4. Consistent Wake-Up Times

While bedtime consistency matters, many experts say that waking up at the same time daily is even more crucial. Your body sets its internal clock based on that wake-up signal. If you wake up at 6:30 am on weekdays but sleep until 10:00 am on weekends, your Sunday night might be rough as your body tries to handle a shifted schedule.

Alternative: If you want to sleep in a bit on weekends, limit it to about an hour later than your usual weekday rise time. This helps prevent a major "social jet lag" that can throw off your body clock.

5. Daytime Routines and How They Affect Sleep

Your day is not just random hours that happen before bedtime. What you do in the morning and afternoon can impact how you sleep. For example, if you consume caffeine late in the day or take long naps, it might disrupt your night. If you have no break from digital screens all day, you might be overstimulated by bedtime.

Key Daytime Elements

- **Regular Meals**: Having meals at roughly the same times can help regulate your energy levels.
- **Activity Breaks**: Short walks or stretches throughout the day can keep you from feeling restless in the evening.
- **Reduced Evening Stimulants**: Cutting back on caffeine after lunchtime helps ensure you feel ready for bed at night.

6. Handling Naps Wisely

Napping can be a great tool for people who did not sleep well, but if you nap too long or too late in the day, it might push your bedtime back. Generally, a short nap (20 to 30 minutes) early in the afternoon is least likely to disturb your night. Longer naps or late-afternoon naps can reduce nighttime tiredness.

Less-Known Tip: Some people benefit from a "coffee nap," where they drink a small cup of coffee right before a short nap. By the time they wake up, the caffeine starts to kick in. However, this is best done at least 6 or more hours before bed, so it does not interfere with nighttime rest.

7. Evening Wind-Down Activities

We touched on bedtime routines, but let's explore more possible wind-down activities:

1. **Gentle Stretching**: Loosen tight muscles, especially if you sit all day.

2. **Puzzles or Coloring**: Quiet activities that keep your hands busy and mind relaxed.
3. **Listening to Calm Audio**: Soft music or nature sounds at low volume.
4. **Light Chores**: Simple tasks like washing a few dishes or preparing clothes for tomorrow can signal your mind to close out the day. Just avoid anything too stressful or physically intense.

The main idea is to pick activities that do not raise your heart rate or worry you. Avoid heated arguments, scary movies, or intense games right before bed, as they can spark alertness or unease.

8. The Role of Consistent Cues

We often think about routines for babies and kids—bedtime stories, lullabies, and so on. But adults can also benefit from consistent cues. If each night you follow the same steps, your brain starts recognizing the pattern. By the time you reach the final step (like turning off the lamp or lying on the pillow a certain way), your mind has already begun shifting into rest mode.

9. Bedtime and Pets

If you have pets, their routines might affect yours. A dog might need a walk or some time to settle. Cats may roam or meow at night if not given a steady routine. Try to feed pets and give them attention well before your own bedtime routine starts. This way, they are calmer and less likely to disturb you.

Less-Known Tip: For dogs that sleep in the same room, a short, predictable "potty break" right before you begin your bedtime routine can help prevent late-night interruptions.

10. Social Media and Late-Night Communication

Staying in touch with friends or family late at night can disrupt your routine. Even if you enjoy chatting, your body might not, especially if these interactions are lively. It can be helpful to set a "communication curfew," letting people know that after a certain time, you will not be replying until morning. This helps you avoid the temptation to check your phone for messages.

11. Special Considerations for Shift Workers or Irregular Schedules

A strict 9-to-5 schedule is not possible for everyone. If you work rotating shifts, try to keep as much routine as you can. For instance, on night shifts, you might still have a "bedtime routine" in the morning when you get home. You would dim lights or use blackout curtains to mimic nighttime. The key is to keep the steps consistent, even though your "night" might be someone else's daytime.

Less-Known Tip: If your shift changes weekly or monthly, it can be tough to maintain a stable schedule. Focus on small anchors, like specific routines for meals and hygiene, that do not change, even if the time of day does.

12. What to Do If You Stray from the Routine

Life happens. You might stay out late for a friend's event or have a family emergency that wakes you at odd hours. Missing a routine for one or two nights will not ruin your overall rest if you return to normal as soon as possible. The body can handle small disruptions. Just do not let it become a long-term pattern if you can help it.

Practical Approach: If you stay up several hours past your usual bedtime one night, do not try to "sleep until noon" the next day to make up for it. That could make your schedule bounce around more. Instead, return to your normal wake-up time or at least limit the extra sleep to an hour. Then, let your body readjust the following night.

13. Keeping the Routine Interesting

Some fear that a daily routine might become dull. You can still have variety within the structure. For example, you might always start winding down around

9:30 pm, but some nights you stretch while listening to soft music, while other nights you do a bit of coloring or read a short story. The key is maintaining the same overall timeline, even if the exact activities change.

14. The Power of Mini-Routines During the Day

Beyond the main bedtime routine, small habits throughout the day can support stable rest. Examples:

- **Morning Routine**: Waking up at the same time, opening the curtains to let in light, drinking a glass of water, and eating a small breakfast.
- **Lunch Routine**: Eating lunch around the same time, perhaps stepping outside for fresh air.
- **Afternoon Break**: Even a 10-minute break to move around or rest your eyes from screens.
- **Transition from Work to Home**: Changing out of work clothes, planning dinner, and so on.

Each mini-routine helps keep your body and mind in balance, reducing chaotic transitions that can lead to stress or poor rest at night.

15. Combining Routines with Other Sleep Tips

We have covered many topics: environment, light, nutrition, stress, and exercise. A routine weaves these together. For instance:

- **After Dinner**: Dim lights, do some light chores.
- **End of Chores**: Take a warm shower or bath to aid muscle relaxation (as the body cools down afterward, it promotes rest).
- **Screen Curfew**: An hour before bed, put phones away or switch them to night mode.
- **Calm Activity**: Read a printed book or write in a journal.
- **Set the Bedroom**: Adjust the temperature, turn on a small night light if needed.
- **Final Steps**: Lie down and practice a short breathing exercise.

When these steps happen at roughly the same time each evening, your body will start to expect them, making it easier to feel sleepy when the final step arrives.

16. Dealing with Evening Events

Sometimes, you might have a planned gathering, a show, or other social events that run late. In these cases, accept that your bedtime routine will shift for that evening. To limit the disruption:

1. **Plan in Advance**: If you know you will be out late, try to maintain parts of your routine beforehand. For example, dim lights and avoid heavy meals leading up to the event.
2. **Wind Down as Soon as Possible**: The moment you get home, do a shortened version of your usual routine rather than jumping into bed immediately.
3. **Avoid Doing It Often**: If you have events every single night, your routine might never get a chance to stabilize.

17. Children's Routines for Adult Rest

If you have kids, their routines matter for your rest too. A child who goes to bed late or wakes up several times in the night can disrupt your schedule. Families often do best when everyone has some kind of predictable routine. Even teenagers can benefit from a stable bedtime and wake-up time, though they might naturally want to stay up later. Clear rules about electronics, lights, and screen use can help the entire household rest better.

18. Travel and Time Zone Shifts

Travel can throw off your routine, especially if crossing time zones. The best way to adapt is to shift your routine to local time as soon as you can. Get morning light in the new location, eat meals on the local schedule, and try not to nap too much during the day if you arrive tired. This encourages faster alignment with the new time zone.

Less-Known Tip: Melatonin supplements are sometimes used for jet lag, but they are not the only solution. Keeping your usual habits—like a small bedtime snack or reading time—can help your body feel a sense of normalcy in a new place.

19. Tracking Your Routine

If you are unsure how your day flows, a simple log can help. Write down when you woke up, your mealtimes, exercise sessions, and when you started and ended your bedtime routine. After a few weeks, you can spot patterns. Maybe you notice that every time you push dinner past 9:00 pm, you have trouble falling asleep before midnight. Or you see that on days you skip your afternoon walk, you feel restless at bedtime. Adjust your routine based on what you learn.

20. Putting It All into Practice

A good routine can be a game-changer for your rest. It provides a stable framework so your body knows when to be active and when to wind down. Here are the main points to remember:

1. **Set a Target Bedtime**: Choose a realistic time that allows 7 to 9 hours of rest, depending on your needs.
2. **Wake Up Consistently**: Let your body see the same wake-up time most days.
3. **Create a Calming Bedtime Routine**: Include actions that signal rest, like dimming lights, reading, or gentle stretching.
4. **Watch Daytime Habits**: Keep caffeine, naps, and screen usage in check so they do not sabotage your night.
5. **Adapt but Don't Abandon**: Life events may cause you to stray from routine. Return to it as soon as you can.

With a routine, you have a roadmap for your day. Combine it with the tips from earlier chapters—like proper light exposure and a comfortable sleep environment—and you stand a good chance of achieving more restful nights. In the next chapters, we will look at more myths about rest, the connection between mood and sleep, different sleeping positions, and more. Each piece contributes to a fuller picture of how to unlock the best rest possible.

Chapter 11: Sleep Myths

Many ideas about sleep circulate among people. Some of these ideas may have a bit of truth, while others can be misleading or entirely incorrect. Myths about rest can lead to poor habits, added stress, or confusion over what truly helps a person rest well. In this chapter, we will examine a range of beliefs people hold about sleep. We will clarify which ones have strong support, which ones are half-truths, and which ones are not accurate at all. By the end of this chapter, you will be better able to figure out which ideas can help you and which ones might hurt your rest.

1. "Everyone Needs 8 Hours of Sleep"

One of the most common sleep myths is that there is a strict number of hours everyone needs each night, usually stated as exactly eight hours. While eight hours is often given as a general guideline, actual needs vary. Some people function well on seven hours, while others thrive on nine. Teenagers might need even more, and older adults might shift to a slightly shorter rest time, though that is not always the case. The body's signals and how one feels after waking up are often the best clues about personal needs.

Why the Myth Persists

- Rounded numbers are easy to remember.
- Many studies use a range of 7–9 hours for adults, so people often pick the midpoint.
- Some workplaces or cultural norms push the idea that 8 hours is the magic number.

The Reality

- Sleep needs are individual.
- If you feel refreshed on 7 hours, you may not need to push for 8.
- If you are still groggy after 8 hours, you may need a bit more.

2. "Older Adults Only Need 5 or 6 Hours of Sleep"

Another common claim is that older adults naturally require much less rest, such as only 5 or 6 hours a night. While it is true that some changes happen in sleep patterns as people age—like waking up earlier or having a slightly harder time getting long stretches of deep rest—it does not mean older adults do not need enough sleep to feel healthy. Often, they still need around 7 or 8 hours, but they might break it up differently over the night or take brief daytime rests.

Why the Myth Persists

- Observations of older relatives rising earlier in the morning can lead younger people to assume older adults need less rest.
- Age-related conditions can make continuous rest harder, leading to frequent waking.

The Reality

- Many older adults still aim for about 7 or more hours of restful sleep.
- Naps can help, but they do not fully replace a good stretch of nighttime rest.
- If an older person is only getting 5 hours at night, they might be missing important stages of rest and could feel fatigue during the day.

---

3. "Snoring Is Always Harmless"

Snoring is often seen as a normal or even funny trait. While light or occasional snoring can be harmless, loud, frequent snoring can be a warning sign of deeper issues, such as sleep apnea. Sleep apnea involves pauses in breathing and can raise the risk of health problems like high blood pressure or heart trouble. If someone snores loudly and experiences daytime tiredness, it is wise to look into whether there is an underlying condition.

Why the Myth Persists

- Snoring jokes and cartoons treat it as minor.
- Many people snore occasionally (like when they have a cold), which can be harmless.

The Reality

- Persistent loud snoring should not be ignored.
- A partner noticing gasps or choking sounds during sleep could be an indicator of a serious issue.
- Checking with a health professional is the best step if snoring is heavy and frequent.

---

4. "Sleeping Extra on Weekends Makes Up for Poor Sleep"

People often try to catch up on rest by sleeping a lot on weekends. While you may feel a temporary boost, it does not fully make up for chronic rest loss. If you regularly sleep poorly on weekdays—getting only 5 or 6 hours a night—and then try to sleep 10 or 11 hours on a weekend, your body may still be dealing with the impact of ongoing rest shortages. Also, sleeping late on weekends can shift your internal clock, making it harder to fall asleep at your usual time on Sunday night.

Why the Myth Persists

- It feels logical that if you have a "sleep debt," you can pay it off by sleeping more on days off.
- People often do feel somewhat better after a catch-up day.

The Reality

- One or two weekend "sleep binges" may help a little, but they will not fully fix a long-term habit of not sleeping enough.
- It is more helpful to keep a steady nightly schedule with enough hours.

---

5. "If You Wake Up in the Middle of the Night, You Should Stay in Bed Until You Fall Asleep Again"

Many people believe they must stay in bed no matter how long they are lying awake. However, if you are tossing and turning for more than about 15 or 20 minutes, it might help to get out of bed for a short while. A short, quiet activity like reading a light (non-stressful) book in dim light can help shift the mind away from worry. Then, once you feel sleepy again, you can return to bed. Staying in bed awake for long stretches can build an uneasy connection in the mind between your bed and restlessness.

Why the Myth Persists

- People think bed is the "only place" to fall asleep, so they wait there, hoping it will happen quickly.
- A fear of losing more rest time can lead them to stay put, even if they are anxious or frustrated.

The Reality

- Sometimes leaving the bed for a bit and doing a calm activity in low light helps break the cycle of tension.
- Returning to bed when the body is actually feeling sleepy can speed up the process of drifting off.

---

6. "Naps Are Always Bad for Your Nighttime Sleep"

Some believe that naps always ruin nighttime rest. While it is true that long or late naps can make it harder to sleep at night, short and well-timed naps (usually in the early afternoon for about 20–30 minutes) can boost energy without harming nighttime sleep. The key is to keep naps brief and not too late in the day. This way, you will not mess up the body's natural drive to rest at your normal bedtime.

Why the Myth Persists

- Some individuals do feel wide awake at bedtime after a poorly timed or lengthy nap.
- Negative experiences from a single, long nap can lead to generalizing that all naps are harmful.

The Reality

- Controlled naps can be helpful, especially if you are truly short on rest.
- It is best to experiment and see if short naps help you feel better or if they disrupt your nighttime rest.

7. "You Can Function Perfectly on 4 or 5 Hours of Sleep if You Train Yourself"

There are stories about famous people who claim to sleep only a few hours a night and still do fine. While there might be very rare cases of individuals with genetic traits that allow them to function on significantly less rest, most people cannot simply "train" themselves to need less. Over time, chronic lack of rest often leads to higher stress, poor focus, mood swings, and other health risks.

Why the Myth Persists

- People look up to high achievers and assume they can copy their habits, including short rest times.
- Some individuals can push through with caffeine and adrenaline, masking tiredness for a while.

The Reality

- Most adults need at least 7 hours of good rest to perform their best.
- Forcing yourself to get by on 4 or 5 hours can lead to serious health problems over time.

8. "Alcohol Before Bed Helps You Sleep Better"

Some folks drink alcohol at night to feel relaxed and fall asleep. While it might make you drowsy initially, alcohol actually disrupts the later parts of the sleep cycle. It can cause you to wake up after a few hours, lead to bathroom visits, or reduce the quality of deeper rest stages. Also, alcohol can worsen breathing problems, such as snoring or sleep apnea.

Why the Myth Persists

- The initial sedative effect of alcohol gives a false impression of improved rest.
- Some cultures encourage a nightcap as a way to "wind down."

The Reality

- Alcohol disrupts sleep architecture, the normal pattern of sleep stages.
- You might wake up feeling groggy or dehydrated, which cancels any benefits of falling asleep faster.

---

9. "Watching TV in Bed Helps You Relax"

Many people like to watch TV in bed, thinking it is a good way to unwind. However, the bright screen light—along with the engaging or dramatic content—can stimulate your brain, making it harder to doze off. Even if you feel like you can drift off with the TV on, the quality of rest might be reduced because background noise or sudden changes in light can pull you out of deeper stages.

Why the Myth Persists

- TV often feels comforting or entertaining, which might temporarily reduce worry.
- People confuse the feeling of "zoning out" in front of the TV with genuine rest.

The Reality

- The mind can remain slightly alert due to movement, noise, and flickering light.
- It is better to watch TV in another room, then move to bed once you are ready for lights-out.

---

10. "Exercising at Night Ruins Sleep"

It is sometimes said that if you exercise at night, you will be too energized to rest. In reality, it depends on the type and timing of the workout. Very intense training right before bed can indeed increase heart rate and body temperature, delaying rest. But a moderate or light session earlier in the evening—like yoga, a casual walk, or gentle stretching—can help you relax and potentially lead to better rest. The key is to finish high-intensity workouts a couple of hours before bedtime if possible.

Why the Myth Persists

- People notice they feel "pumped up" after vigorous exercise, so they assume all evening activity is harmful.
- Some advice lumps all exercise together without considering intensity or timing.

The Reality

- Mild or moderate nighttime workouts can be helpful for certain individuals.
- Pay attention to your personal response. If a late workout keeps you awake, move it earlier.

---

11. "If You Cannot Sleep, You Should Just Lie There Until Morning"

Some people believe that if they wake at 3:00 am and cannot go back to sleep, they should remain in bed with eyes closed until the alarm rings. While lying calmly might help you rest a bit, the frustration of not actually sleeping can build up. Sometimes, getting out of bed to do a quiet, non-stimulating task (like flipping through a simple magazine or doing slow breathing in a dimly lit room) can help reset your mind. Then you can try sleeping again.

Why the Myth Persists

- Fear of "missing out" on potential sleep makes people not want to leave the bed.
- Lack of alternative ideas for what to do if they cannot fall back asleep.

The Reality

- Briefly getting up can break the cycle of irritation or anxious thoughts.
- Returning to bed when feeling at least somewhat drowsy can improve the chance of falling asleep again.

12. "You Shouldn't Wake Sleepwalkers"

A popular myth is that it is dangerous to wake a sleepwalker, and it is better to let them walk around or guide them back to bed. While startling a sleepwalker could cause confusion or a temporary fright, letting them wander can be even riskier. They could hurt themselves by bumping into furniture, falling down stairs, or leaving the house.

Why the Myth Persists

- Widespread tales mention that waking a sleepwalker can cause them shock or even severe harm.
- Fiction and movies have perpetuated this idea.

The Reality

- If you find someone sleepwalking, it is best to gently direct them away from danger or carefully wake them if necessary.
- Yes, they might be disoriented, but that is better than allowing them to roam unsafely.

---

13. "Sleeping Pills Are the Only Way to Fix Serious Sleep Problems"

While medications can help in certain cases, especially if prescribed by a professional, they are often not the sole or best long-term solution for ongoing rest troubles. Many sleep problems can be improved through changes in habits, environment, stress management, or therapy techniques. Pills might be useful for short-term or severe issues, but relying on them without trying other methods can lead to side effects, tolerance, or dependence.

Why the Myth Persists

- Quick fixes are appealing in today's busy world.
- Advertising might lead some to believe pills are the simplest answer.

The Reality

- Cognitive methods, better habits, and changes to daily routines can address root causes.

- Medication has its place, but it should not be the only plan for most long-term issues.

---

14. "All Sleep Disorders Are the Same and Have the Same Solutions"

People sometimes lump sleep problems under one label. The truth is that insomnia, sleep apnea, restless legs, circadian rhythm issues, and other conditions each have different causes and approaches. One-size-fits-all solutions rarely work. For instance, a person with apnea might need a breathing device, while someone with restless legs might need to adjust diet or iron levels. Getting a proper diagnosis is key to finding the right fix.

Why the Myth Persists

- General tips like "get more rest" or "avoid screens at night" are repeated so often that people assume they handle all types of problems.
- Lack of awareness that certain conditions have distinct signs.

The Reality

- If standard tips do not help, it might be time to see a specialist.
- Each condition can need a unique blend of changes, gadgets, or therapies.

---

15. "Only Lazy People Nap or Sleep More Than 8 Hours"

Some folks assume that anyone who naps or sleeps longer than the typical range is lazy. This belief can cause guilt for those who truly need extra rest or who benefit from short midday rests. Different life stages (like growth phases in teens or healing after illness) can require additional rest. Also, certain schedules or physical demands might lead some people to need a nap.

Why the Myth Persists

- Cultural norms in certain places label naps as unproductive.
- Social media might show high achievers functioning on little sleep, which some mistake as the standard.

The Reality

- Sleep needs differ. Some people truly need more than 8 hours to feel strong during the day.
- Napping can enhance productivity if done properly.

---

16. "A Couple of Nights of Bad Sleep Means You Have Insomnia"

Insomnia is characterized by ongoing trouble falling or staying asleep, often lasting for weeks or months. A single difficult night or even a brief stretch of poor rest caused by stress, travel, or a minor illness does not necessarily mean you have clinical insomnia. Many people jump to the conclusion that having trouble for a few nights is a permanent problem, which might create more anxiety and actually make falling asleep harder.

Why the Myth Persists

- The word "insomnia" is sometimes used loosely to describe any trouble sleeping.
- People can panic when they cannot sleep, assuming the worst.

The Reality

- True insomnia is typically a longer-term condition.
- Occasional poor nights are normal and can often be fixed with simple measures like reducing stress or adjusting the sleep environment.

---

17. "Waking Up at Night Is Always a Sign of a Problem"

Some individuals worry that any nighttime waking is bad. In fact, it can be normal to have brief awakenings, especially at the end of a sleep cycle. You might turn over, adjust your blanket, and go back to sleep without much trouble. As long as you do not lie awake for extended periods, this is often not a big issue. However, if you are awake for 30 minutes or more multiple times each night, or you feel very tired the next day, it could indicate a concern.

Why the Myth Persists

- A strong belief exists that healthy rest is always unbroken.
- People assume they must sleep like a log from bedtime to morning.

The Reality

- Short, minor awakenings can be normal for many.
- If awakenings are frequent or you feel unrested, examine possible stress or environmental triggers.

---

18. "Dreams Are Meaningless" or "Dreams Always Predict the Future"

Dreams stir a lot of debate. Some think they are pointless brain noise, while others believe they hold deep secrets or can foretell events. The truth is likely somewhere in the middle. Dreams often reflect our daily thoughts, emotions, or memories. They can be shaped by stress, hopes, or experiences. While they usually do not predict the future, they can reveal feelings you might be sorting through.

Why the Myth Persists

- Dreams are personal and can sometimes line up with real-life events, encouraging superstition.
- Various cultural stories about dreams shape how we see them.

The Reality

- Dreams are part of the mind's activity during REM sleep.
- They can offer insights into emotions, but they do not always have a clear or fixed meaning.

---

19. "You Can Drink as Much Caffeine as You Want if You're Tired"

Some people believe that if they are sleepy, they can consume unlimited coffee, energy drinks, or tea to counteract fatigue. However, too much caffeine can lead to restlessness, jitters, and difficulty sleeping at night. It may mask your tiredness for a short time, but the underlying cause—lack of rest—remains. Also, large amounts of caffeine can linger in the body for hours, making it harder to have a full night of good rest.

Why the Myth Persists

- Quick energy boosts feel good in the moment.
- Caffeine is widely accepted and easy to access.

The Reality

- A moderate amount of caffeine in the morning can be fine for most people.
- Going overboard or drinking it late can trap you in a cycle of low energy and poor rest.

---

20. Final Thoughts on Myths

Misunderstandings about sleep can keep you from addressing real issues or lead you to adopt unhelpful habits. Being aware of the facts helps you avoid these pitfalls. If you are dealing with a rest problem and find yourself repeating a common piece of advice, stop and check if it is a myth or if it actually applies to you. The more you learn about actual sleep science, the more likely you are to spot half-truths and avoid them.

Key Points

- Many popular claims about rest do not hold up under closer inspection.
- Individual differences matter—one-size-fits-all ideas can lead you astray.
- "Quick fixes" like weekend catch-up sleep or heavy reliance on caffeine do not solve deeper issues.
- When in doubt, see a qualified professional, especially for ongoing or severe problems.

The next chapter will focus on how sleep and mood interact. Many people notice changes in their mood after just one poor night of rest, and ongoing low rest can raise the risk of serious emotional challenges. We will look at why this link exists and what can be done to protect both rest and mental well-being.

Chapter 12: Sleep and Mood

Mood and sleep share a strong connection. You might have noticed that after a rough night, you feel irritated or down the next day. People who regularly lack rest often show higher levels of sadness, worry, or anger. Similarly, if you are in a poor mood, you may find it harder to rest well because worries or negative thoughts keep your mind active. Understanding the ways that rest and emotional states affect each other can help you protect both your emotional health and your rest quality.

Below, we will look at how rest affects mood at both short-term and long-term levels. We will also discuss how mood challenges, such as long-lasting sadness or severe worry, can harm sleep. By the end of this chapter, you will have ideas on how to keep a stable emotional state that supports restful nights, and ways to adjust your habits if you notice stress creeping in.

1. How a Single Poor Night Affects Mood

Just one night of bad rest can change how you feel the next day. You might notice yourself:

- Feeling more annoyed by small problems.
- Lacking energy or interest in daily tasks.
- Finding it hard to focus or learn new things.
- Snapping at friends or family.

These changes arise because rest is linked to how the brain manages emotions and attention. When the brain does not get the time it needs to reset, it can react more strongly to minor setbacks.

2. Ongoing Poor Sleep and Emotional Health

When rest troubles become chronic, the effects on mood can deepen. People can develop ongoing irritability, gloominess, or even hopelessness. Over time, these mood shifts can lead to social or work problems, such as arguments with loved ones or poor performance on the job, which can add more stress and further hurt rest. This can spiral into a loop: the worse you feel, the harder it is to rest, and the less you rest, the worse your mood becomes.

---

3. Stress and Worries

Stress about work, finances, or relationships can make you feel tense. We discussed stress in an earlier chapter, but here we focus on how mood issues from stress can keep you awake. When the mind is tense, it is harder to shift into a calm state needed for sleep. Instead, thoughts might race, or you may dwell on the day's problems.

Tips to Break This Cycle

- Keep a notebook by the bed to write down any tasks or concerns so they are not swirling in your head.
- Practice a short relaxation method, such as gentle breathing or muscle loosening, to reduce stress chemicals in the body before bed.
- Speak with someone you trust, or seek professional advice if stress is extreme.

---

4. Low Mood and Clinical Sadness

Feeling sad from time to time is normal. But when sadness is strong and lasts for weeks or more, it might signal deeper emotional problems. One of the core signs of ongoing sadness is trouble with rest: sleeping too much or too little. People who feel very sad might struggle to fall asleep or might wake up in the early morning feeling hopeless. Alternatively, some might sleep all day, lacking the desire to get up.

Why Sadness Disrupts Sleep

- The body's chemical balance shifts. Certain chemicals that help with motivation and energy can become low.
- Thoughts about negative feelings can fill the mind at bedtime.

- Disturbed daily routines can lead to irregular bedtimes and wake times, making sleep less stable.

If you suspect you have lasting sadness that affects rest, consider talking to a mental health professional. They can help you learn strategies to manage negative thoughts and regulate sleep patterns.

5. Worry and Sleep

Worry is marked by excessive thoughts about future events or potential problems. People who worry a lot might lie in bed trying to plan for every possible outcome of a situation, such as a test, a meeting, or personal issues. This mental overload can cause trouble falling asleep or cause frequent awakenings.

Methods to Handle Worry

- Set a "worry time" earlier in the day. Give yourself permission to list concerns or try problem-solving for 15 minutes in the afternoon, so it is not all stored up for bedtime.
- Use calm focus methods—like counting breaths or visualizing simple, steady images—to push away ongoing mental chatter.
- If worry remains severe over time, consider seeking counseling or therapy that offers specialized skills to reduce anxious thoughts.

6. The Cycle of Anger and Rest

Anger can also block good rest. If you go to bed feeling resentful or upset, your body may still be keyed up. Heart rate can be higher, muscles can be tense, and your mind can replay arguments or insults. Breaking out of anger before bed can involve:

- Practicing a simple reflection on what went right during the day.
- Letting yourself close the day's conflict by making a plan to address it tomorrow instead of mulling it over all night.
- Using calming stretches, gentle yoga poses, or slow breathing to bring heart rate and muscle tension down.

7. Hormones That Connect Mood and Sleep

Your body has certain chemicals that regulate mood and rest, such as serotonin, dopamine, and cortisol. When rest is poor, the levels and timing of these chemicals may shift. For example, cortisol might stay high if you are under stress, making you feel uneasy and jumpy at night. Serotonin, involved in feeling content, can be thrown off by chronic rest loss or mental distress. This means that both the emotional state and the rest cycle can be affected by the same biological factors.

---

8. The Role of REM in Processing Emotions

During rapid eye movement (REM) sleep, the brain is active and processes a lot of the day's experiences, including emotional ones. Dreams often arise here, and they can be tied to our deepest worries or hopes. A healthy amount of REM might help the brain "file away" emotional experiences, leading to more stable moods the next day. If you are not reaching enough REM (perhaps due to constant interruptions or substances like alcohol), you might miss out on this important nightly processing.

---

9. Mood Disorders and Sleep Disorders

Mood disorders, such as ongoing sadness or severe worry, often coincide with certain rest disorders:

- **Insomnia**: People with a low or anxious mood may have trouble initiating or maintaining rest.
- **Hypersomnia**: Some with strong sadness may sleep excessively but still feel unrefreshed.
- **Disturbed Circadian Rhythms**: Irregular mood can lead to inconsistent bedtimes and wake times, throwing off the internal clock.

It can be a chicken-and-egg problem: does poor mood cause poor rest, or does poor rest cause poor mood? Often, it is both. Addressing both sides at once can help.

10. Social Impact and Isolation

When you are in a poor mood, you might withdraw from friends or family. This can lead to reduced social support, which can make you feel more alone and potentially worsen sad or anxious feelings. As this emotional weight grows, rest can suffer even more. On the flip side, good social interactions can boost mood, which can lead to better rest patterns. Regular contact with supportive people often helps break the cycle of emotional upset and poor rest.

---

11. Ways to Boost Mood for Better Rest

a) Gratitude List

Writing down a short list of things that went well or that you appreciate each day can shift your focus. Even on tough days, noting small positives (like a warm meal or a kind message from someone) can reduce negative thought loops at bedtime.

b) Light Exposure

As discussed, sunlight helps regulate the body's internal clock. It also has a positive effect on mood for many people. Aim for some daylight exposure, even if briefly, to help stabilize both rest and mental well-being.

c) Routine

We explored the power of routine in the previous chapter. A steady daily pattern helps keep the mind from becoming chaotic. When your day is organized, you feel more in control, which can ease worries.

d) Movement

Regular activity, even a short daily walk, can reduce tension and lift mood. This can help you relax at night.

12. Foods and Mood

There are foods that seem to help stabilize mood, including those with complex carbs, protein, healthy fats, vitamins, and minerals. On the other hand, large amounts of sugar or heavy junk food can cause spikes and crashes in energy, possibly affecting mood and rest. Staying hydrated is also important, as dehydration can lead to irritability and fatigue.

13. Screen Time and Emotional Health

Looking at social media or stressful news late at night can trigger emotional upset. Disagreements online or seeing negative headlines can keep your mind buzzing. Even if you do not engage in arguments, the content might linger in your thoughts. Turning off screens at least 30 to 60 minutes before bed can protect both your rest and your emotional calm.

14. Signs You Might Need Extra Help

- Feeling sad, hopeless, or worried most days for longer than two weeks.
- Trouble sleeping that persists despite making changes to routine and environment.
- Loss of interest in hobbies or activities you once enjoyed.
- Finding it impossible to relax at bedtime, no matter what you try.
- Thoughts of self-harm or extreme hopelessness.

If any of these are present, contacting a mental health professional could be beneficial. They can offer therapy, guidance, or other options that target both your emotional health and your rest.

15. The Benefits of Therapy and Counseling

Various forms of therapy can support both mood and rest. One example is a type of talk therapy that helps you adjust unhelpful thought patterns and behaviors. There are also specific programs that combine therapy with rest-focused ideas to break cycles of worry at bedtime. You do not have to face mood and rest issues alone; trained counselors can teach you proven skills.

16. Mind Practices for Calmness

a) Breathing Drills

Simple approaches, like inhaling through the nose for a few seconds, holding for a moment, then exhaling slowly through the mouth, can calm the body's stress response.

b) Progressive Tension Release

Tighten and then release muscle groups, from your feet to your head. This helps the body let go of tension that can keep you awake.

c) Imagery

Picture a place that feels calm—maybe a meadow or a gentle beach scene. Focus on small details in your mind: the sounds, textures, and colors. This can help push out negative or stressful thoughts.

---

17. Breaking Negative Thought Loops

When you are in bed with swirling thoughts about daily worries or self-criticism, try these steps:

1. **Acknowledge the Thought**: Do not fight it too hard. Name it: "I am worrying about tomorrow's meeting."
2. **Shift Attention**: Move to something neutral—like counting your breaths or noticing the coolness of the sheets.
3. **Repeat as Needed**: If the thought returns, calmly redirect your focus again. This takes practice but can improve with time.

---

18. Mood, Sleep, and Physical Health

Poor rest can raise the risk of various physical issues, including heart problems, weight changes, and more. A low mood can also lower motivation to exercise or eat well, which in turn can make it even harder to sleep well. By spotting the link between mood, rest, and physical health, you can address multiple areas at once. For instance, committing to moderate daily exercise not only helps your heart but can lift mood and support rest.

19. Social Support and Group Activities

Finding a social setting—like a local group for walking, a community class, or just meeting a friend for a shared hobby—can help break the pattern of negative mood leading to restless nights. Shared laughter, mild physical activity, or even calm social bonding can reduce stress hormones, making it easier to rest at the end of the day.

20. Bringing It All Together

Mood and rest are partners: each one influences the other. A single poor night can lead to a cranky or sad day, and a string of tough days can lead to ongoing rest problems. Here is how you can keep them in balance:

1. **Stay Aware**: Watch for signs that your mood is slipping or that you are having trouble resting.
2. **Act Early**: Use stress reduction or mood-supporting habits before problems grow bigger.
3. **Seek Help**: If sadness, worry, or anger feels unmanageable, talk to a professional.
4. **Use Healthy Habits**: Regular exercise, solid nutrition, light management, and a stable routine all help keep your mood steadier.
5. **Limit Late Stimuli**: Avoid intense social media, TV, or arguments right before bed.

Managing your emotional state will make it easier to sleep soundly. Similarly, making sure you rest enough each night helps keep your mood on a steady path. Both matter for a complete sense of well-being. In the next chapters, we will explore other parts of rest, such as sleeping positions, the art of napping, and ways to shift how you think about rest overall—each of these is a vital part of forming a complete plan for better nights and brighter days.

Chapter 13: Sleeping Positions

We have covered many things that affect how well a person sleeps: stress, environment, light, and more. Now let's look at how the way you lie down can impact the quality of rest. Many people do not think much about this. They assume everyone just picks whichever position feels right. But the truth is, certain positions can help or hurt depending on personal needs. In this chapter, we will explore the main sleeping positions, their pros and cons, and ways to make each one more comfortable. We will also look at special cases, such as sleeping while expecting a baby or dealing with particular aches. By the end, you should have a clearer idea of how to position your body for a calmer, more refreshing sleep.

1. The Basics of Body Alignment

When you lie down, the alignment of your head, neck, spine, and hips matters. If one area is twisted or strained, you could wake up with aches, tingling, or general discomfort. Over time, poor alignment can contribute to ongoing back or neck problems. Paying attention to posture in bed can be as important as good posture when standing or sitting.

Key Points

- Your spine has a natural curve. A position that flattens or exaggerates that curve can cause stress on muscles and nerves.
- A mattress that is too soft might let your body sink in deeply, throwing off alignment. A very hard mattress can create pressure points.
- Proper pillow support is crucial, as it keeps the neck in line with the rest of your spine.

2. Main Sleeping Positions

Most people switch positions during the night. However, they often have a go-to posture that they return to. Let's look at the main ones:

1. **Back**
2. **Side**
3. **Stomach**
4. **Combination** (moving between at least two positions)

Each has different effects on breathing, digestion, spine health, and comfort.

2.1 Sleeping on Your Back

This position is sometimes called the supine position. It is often recommended by physical therapists because it can help maintain a neutral spine alignment, especially if the right pillow and mattress are used.

Pros

- **Neutral Spine Alignment**: If you have a supportive mattress and a pillow that is not too high, your neck stays in line with the spine.
- **Facial Skin Health**: Your face is not pressed against pillows, which might help reduce certain skin issues.
- **Reduced Wrinkles**: Because your face is not squashed, some people believe it might help minimize lines on the face, though this is a minor point compared to the health benefits.

Cons

- **Snoring and Apnea Worsening**: If you tend to snore or have apnea, lying on your back can make your tongue or soft tissues block the airway more easily.
- **Back Discomfort**: If the lower back arches too much or if the mattress is too stiff or sagging, you can end up with lower back pain.

Tips

- **Pillow Under Knees**: Placing a thin pillow or rolled towel beneath your knees can relieve pressure on the lower spine.
- **Use a Supportive Pillow Under the Head**: You do not want your head tilted too far forward or backward. A medium loft pillow often works for back sleepers.
- **Avoid Thick Pillows**: Overly thick pillows can push the head too far up, straining the neck.

2.2 Sleeping on Your Side

Side sleeping is very common. Many people find it comfortable, especially if they have a pillow that supports the head and helps keep the spine straight. There are two main side positions: left side and right side. Each can have different effects on body functions.

Pros

- **Less Snoring**: Side sleeping tends to keep the airway more open compared to lying on the back.
- **Digestion**: For some, sleeping on the left side in particular may help reduce acid reflux, since the stomach is located more to the left in the body.
- **Reduced Lower Back Stress**: If done with good support, side sleeping can take strain off the spine.

Cons

- **Shoulder or Hip Pressure**: Lying on one side all night can lead to numbness or pain in the shoulder or hip pressed against the mattress, especially if the mattress is very firm.
- **Neck Misalignment**: If the pillow is too high or too low, the neck might bend awkwardly, leading to stiffness.
- **Facial Compression**: The side of your face is pressed against the pillow, which may lead to temporary lines or mild facial discomfort for some.

Tips

- **Use a Supportive Pillow**: It should fill the gap between your ear and the mattress, keeping your neck in line with your spine.
- **Place a Pillow Between Knees**: This helps align the hips and reduce twisting of the lower spine.
- **Alternate Sides**: If you always lie on one side, you might develop imbalances or shoulder soreness. Switch sides during the night or from night to night.

Left Side vs. Right Side

- **Left Side**: May be better for digestion and reducing heartburn.

- **Right Side**: Some people find it more comfortable for the heart area if they have certain heart conditions, though this can vary.

2.3 Sleeping on Your Stomach

Stomach sleeping, also called the prone position, is generally not recommended by many health professionals. It can strain the neck and lower back. However, some individuals find it the only way they can doze off.

Pros

- **Reduced Snoring**: In some cases, lying face-down can keep the airway more open than lying on the back.
- **Comfort for a Few**: A small number of people with unique conditions might find it helpful.

Cons

- **Neck Twist**: You have to turn your head to one side to breathe, which can strain neck muscles and joints.
- **Spinal Alignment Problems**: Unless you have a very thin pillow or no pillow at all, the spine might curve in unnatural ways, leading to morning pain.
- **Face Pressure**: The face is pressed into the pillow or turned sharply to the side.

Tips

- **Use a Very Thin Pillow**: Reduces the head tilt required. Some stomach sleepers even use no pillow.
- **Small Pillow Under Hips**: This can help reduce the arch in the lower back.
- **Check Mattress**: A sagging mattress can worsen alignment for a stomach sleeper.

2.4 Combination Sleeping

Many people are "combination" sleepers, shifting between two or more positions throughout the night. This can help prevent prolonged pressure on one area of the body. However, it can also mean that you need a mattress and pillow setup that can handle different poses.

Pros

- **Less Pressure Buildup**: You might avoid shoulder, hip, or back pain by moving around.
- **Adaptability**: If one area gets uncomfortable, you naturally switch to another posture.

Cons

- **Pillow Challenges**: A pillow that is perfect for side sleeping might be too high for back sleeping.
- **Frequent Movement**: Waking up multiple times to switch positions can lead to broken rest if you are a very light sleeper.

Tips

- **Adjustable Pillow**: Some pillows allow you to remove or add filling to find a middle ground.
- **Memory Foam or Hybrid Mattress**: These can adapt to various positions by providing support and cushioning.
- **Body Pillow**: Large pillows can help you transition between side and back positions with minimal strain.

---

3. Special Situations

3.1 Sleeping While Expecting a Baby

People who are expecting often find that as the baby grows, lying on the back becomes uncomfortable or even discouraged by some health providers in the later months. Left side sleeping is often recommended, as it supports healthy blood flow. A pregnancy pillow—a large, curved pillow—can help support the belly, back, and hips.

Tips

- **Use Pillows for Support**: Tuck one under the belly and another between the knees if side sleeping.
- **Avoid Lying Flat on the Back** in later stages: The growing baby can press on major blood vessels, reducing circulation.

3.2 Aches, Joint Pain, or Injuries

People with joint pain, arthritis, or past injuries may need to pick positions that reduce stress on problem areas. A side sleeper with hip pain might place a cushion to better support the hip. A back sleeper with lower back pain might find relief in sliding a pillow under the knees.

Professional Advice

- If chronic pain or a specific condition exists, it is always good to check with a medical professional. They can suggest specific pillow placements or posture adjustments.

3.3 Acid Reflux or Heartburn

Sleeping slightly propped up or on the left side can help keep stomach acid down, reducing reflux symptoms. A wedge pillow can raise the upper body slightly. Stacking normal pillows can work in a pinch, but they may shift during the night.

---

4. Mattress and Pillow Choices

Your ideal mattress and pillow often depend on your main posture. A side sleeper might need a softer mattress that cushions the shoulder and hip, while a back sleeper might want medium firmness for stable support. Stomach sleepers often benefit from a slightly firmer mattress so they do not sink in.

Pillow Guidelines

- **Back Sleepers**: A medium-loft pillow is often good.
- **Side Sleepers**: A fuller pillow to fill the space between the head and mattress.
- **Stomach Sleepers**: A thin or no pillow to avoid neck strain.

Trying Out Mattresses

- Testing a mattress in a store is helpful, but also note that a few minutes is not the same as an entire night. Some stores or brands offer trial periods so you can see if it works over time.

---

5. Pillow Position Tricks

1. **Between the Knees**: Good for side sleepers to keep the spine aligned.
2. **Under the Knees**: Helps back sleepers reduce lower back strain.
3. **Under the Belly**: For those expecting, it can keep the belly supported.
4. **Wedge Pillow**: Great for elevating the upper body when dealing with reflux or breathing issues.

---

6. The Link Between Position and Snoring

People with mild snoring might reduce it by sleeping on their side. Devices exist that try to keep a person from rolling onto their back, such as special pillows or small attachments. If snoring is heavy or accompanied by pauses in breathing, it could be sleep apnea. Changing position alone might not fix severe apnea, but it can help some.

---

7. Using Body Pillows

Body pillows (long pillows that can stretch from your shoulders down past your knees) are popular with side sleepers, especially those who toss and turn. They allow you to hug the pillow with your arms while placing one leg over part of it, which can ease pressure on the lower back and hips. This can also help some stomach sleepers shift to a half-side posture, which is less straining on the neck.

---

8. Combination of Ergonomics and Personal Comfort

While experts often recommend certain positions, personal comfort cannot be ignored. If you try to force yourself to sleep in a posture that feels unnatural, it might increase stress and reduce your rest quality. Some folks find that slight tweaks to their favorite position—like adding a small pillow—are enough to balance health advice with comfort.

---

9. Changing a Long-Term Habit

If you have slept in the same position for decades, changing can be tricky. You might start on your back but wake up on your stomach. Here are some methods:

1. **Pillow Support**: Place pillows around you to discourage rolling into unwanted positions.
2. **Gradual Adjustment**: Try partial changes, like sleeping on a slight incline if you are used to lying flat on your back.
3. **Consistency**: Keep placing yourself in the new position each night. Over time, the body might adapt.

---

10. Additional Factors Affecting Sleep Posture

- **Room Temperature**: If it is too hot or cold, you may shift around more often.
- **Nighttime Clothing**: Tight or bunched-up clothes might make certain positions uncomfortable.
- **Bed Sharing**: If you share the bed, your partner's position or movements can affect yours. Also, pets on the bed might cause you to contort to avoid them.

11. Myths About Sleeping Positions

Myth 1: You Should Never Sleep on Your Stomach

- While it is generally not advised for spinal alignment, some people do it without problems, especially if they use certain pillow strategies. Everyone is different.

Myth 2: The Best Position Is the Same for Everyone

- There is no single universal best posture. It depends on personal needs, health issues, and comfort.

Myth 3: Changing Your Primary Position Is Easy

- For some, it can be a slow process requiring mindful efforts and pillow placement.

---

12. Sleep Positions and Breathing Problems

If you have mild breathing problems or nasal congestion, some positions can help open the airways. Slightly propping the upper body on pillows or a wedge can reduce nasal stuffiness for some people. Side lying can also assist in draining sinuses. If breathing issues are severe, it is wise to see a professional who might suggest treatments or special pillow setups.

---

13. Signs You Might Need a Posture Adjustment

- **Frequent Morning Stiffness**: If your neck or back feels tight each morning, alignment might be off.
- **Numbness or Tingling in Arms or Hands**: Could be due to nerve compression from a position that twists or puts pressure on certain spots.
- **Shoulder Pain**: If you are a side sleeper, your mattress or pillow might be too hard or too soft.
- **Frequent Waking**: If you notice you are waking many times to shift position, it might mean discomfort is preventing you from staying in one place.

14. Small Exercises for Bedtime

Sometimes stretching or simple floor exercises before lying down can loosen tight muscles, making any position more comfortable:

- **Knee to Chest**: Gently pull one knee toward your chest, hold, then switch legs.
- **Cat-Camel** (on hands and knees): Gently round the back up (like a frightened cat) and then lower it (like a camel hump).
- **Shoulder Rolls**: While sitting on the edge of the bed, rotate shoulders forward and backward to reduce tension.

These gentle movements can help the body relax and ease into a good posture more naturally.

---

15. Using a Recliner or Adjustable Bed

Some people find that lying flat is not best for them. They might use a recliner or an adjustable bed that lifts the head and sometimes the legs. This can help with circulation, breathing, or back comfort. However, adjustable beds can be costly, and not everyone finds them necessary. If you have special conditions—like severe reflux or certain heart or lung issues—an adjustable setup could offer real benefits.

---

16. Children and Sleep Position

Kids often flop around in all sorts of poses. Generally, younger bodies are more flexible, and parents only need to intervene if the child's position leads to frequent aches or if they have a condition like ear infections or reflux. For most children, letting them settle into a natural posture is fine. Encouraging them to avoid stomach sleeping might be wise if they complain of neck pain. Otherwise, their bodies often guide them to what works best.

17. Travel and Different Beds

When traveling, you might face hotel beds, unfamiliar pillows, or even sleeping on a couch at a relative's house. Being aware of your posture needs can help you adapt:

- **Bring Your Own Pillow**: If you have space, a familiar pillow can keep your neck supported in the usual way.
- **Use Towels as Extra Support**: If the mattress is too soft or hard, rolling up towels to place under knees or hips can mimic your home setup.
- **Experiment with Position**: Sometimes in a strange bed, a different posture might be more comfortable.

---

18. Listening to Your Body

Pay attention to how you feel in the morning. If you are frequently stiff, it might be time to consider if the position (or the mattress, or the pillows) is not working. Checking in on how you feel after naps can also reveal if posture is the culprit. A small tweak—like adjusting pillow height—can sometimes make a big difference.

---

19. Position and Temperature Regulation

Some positions might make you feel hotter. For instance, if you are lying on your stomach in very warm blankets, you might build up extra body heat. Side sleeping can allow more air circulation around your torso. If overheating at night is a problem, consider a lighter blanket, cooler room temperature, or moisture-wicking sheets. Then see if you can find a pose that balances comfort with air flow.

---

20. Putting It All Together

Your sleeping position can have a real impact on how refreshed you feel in the morning. While some positions are often considered healthier (back or side), personal preference, specific health needs, and comfort also play huge roles. By tuning in to your body's signals, experimenting with pillows or angles, and choosing the right mattress, you can find a posture that supports restful, comfortable nights.

Key Points

1. **Alignment Is Critical**: The spine, neck, and hips should be in a neutral position as much as possible.
2. **Side and Back Sleeping**: Often recommended for most people, but fine-tune your pillow setup.
3. **Stomach Sleeping**: Not the first choice for many, but if it works for you, use thin pillows to reduce strain.
4. **Small Adjustments Help**: Pillows under knees, between legs, or hugging a body pillow can make a big difference.
5. **Check for Pain**: Regular aches may signal the need to shift positions or upgrade bedding.

Experiment little by little. If you normally wake up with tight muscles, try a slight change, like a better pillow or adding one between your knees. See if your rest improves. Over time, you might find the position that best allows you to drift off and stay asleep without nagging soreness or frequent awakenings. In the next chapter, we will focus on another part of nightly rest: napping. Though not everyone naps, short daytime rests can either boost or hinder nighttime sleep, depending on how and when they are done. We will share insights on using naps wisely to support better overall rest.

Chapter 14: Napping

In the previous chapter, we examined how different sleeping positions can shape the quality of a night's rest. Now we turn to a topic that sometimes sparks debate: napping. For some, naps are a cherished midday break that helps them recharge. For others, naps disrupt nighttime rest. We will explore who might benefit from naps, the ideal nap length and timing, the science behind short rests, and ways to handle common nap-related problems. By the end, you will have a sense of whether naps fit into your daily life and how to make them work (or decide to skip them) without undermining your main night's sleep.

1. What Is a Nap?

A nap is a short period of rest taken during the day, typically lasting from a few minutes up to a couple of hours. Naps can be planned (such as a routine midday rest) or unplanned (when you nod off because you are very tired). Some cultures have a tradition of midday rests, while others see napping as unusual or unproductive.

2. Why People Nap

1. **Energy Slump**: Many people experience a dip in alertness after lunch (often called the "post-lunch dip"). A short rest can help re-energize.
2. **Insufficient Nighttime Sleep**: If you do not get enough rest at night, you might nap to make it through the day.
3. **Shift Work**: Those who work nights might nap during the day to supplement their core sleep.
4. **Cultural or Personal Habit**: Some regions have a normal midday break.
5. **Health Reasons**: Certain conditions or medications can cause fatigue, making naps more common or necessary.

3. Types of Naps

3.1 The Power Nap (10–20 Minutes)

A quick 10–20 minute snooze is often called a power nap. It can give a small boost in alertness and focus without leaving you feeling groggy afterward. You typically stay in lighter stages of rest. This helps you wake up feeling relatively refreshed.

Pros

- Quick recharge.
- Less disruption to nighttime rest if done early enough in the day.

Cons

- Not enough if you are heavily sleep-deprived.
- Some people might still feel a bit disoriented if they are not used to short sleeps.

3.2 The Mid-Length Nap (30–60 Minutes)

A nap around half an hour to an hour may allow you to reach deeper stages of rest. That can help restore energy levels more than a short power nap. However, if you wake up during a deeper stage, you could experience "sleep inertia," meaning you feel groggy for a while.

Pros

- Can be more restful if you are short on night sleep.
- May improve mood and cognitive function for a few hours.

Cons

- Higher chance of grogginess upon waking if you interrupt a deep stage.
- Might risk harming nighttime sleep if done too late in the day.

3.3 The Longer Nap (90+ Minutes)

A nap of 90 minutes or more might include a full sleep cycle, reaching both deep rest and possibly a bit of REM. This could leave you feeling quite refreshed, but it also has a bigger chance of interfering with your usual bedtime.

Pros

- Can help if you have a big sleep debt or need significant rest.
- Might reduce irritability and sharpen thinking for the rest of the day.

Cons

- Might lead to difficulties falling asleep at night, especially if taken late.
- Higher chance of sleep inertia if you wake during a deep stage.

---

4. The Science of Napping

4.1 Brain Waves and Stages

During short naps (under 30 minutes), you mostly stay in lighter stages (Stage N1 and Stage N2). You may not reach deep Stage N3 or REM. Longer naps might allow deeper stages, but that also means a higher risk of grogginess if your alarm rings in the middle of it.

4.2 Circadian Rhythm

Your circadian rhythm influences how alert or sleepy you feel. Around midday or early afternoon, many people naturally have a slight drop in energy. Naps taken at this time may fit with the body's rhythm. A late-afternoon or evening nap, however, might push your bedtime later or reduce the depth of your nighttime sleep.

---

5. How to Nap Wisely

1. **Keep It Short**: If you only need a little boost, aim for about 20 minutes. This helps you avoid deep stages that might cause grogginess.

2. **Consider the Timing**: Early to mid-afternoon is usually best. Napping too late (like after 4:00 or 5:00 pm) can make it harder to fall asleep at night.
3. **Set an Alarm**: If you are worried about oversleeping, use a timer or alarm. This helps stick to the chosen nap length.
4. **Create a Calm Setting**: A quiet, slightly cool space can improve nap quality. If you are at work, maybe find a lounge or use earplugs.
5. **Experiment**: Not everyone's body reacts the same way. Try different lengths and times to see what leaves you feeling best, both right after and at bedtime.

---

6. The "Coffee Nap" Concept

A "coffee nap" means drinking a small cup of coffee right before a short nap. Caffeine takes about 15–20 minutes to start working in most people. By the time you wake up from a 20-minute rest, the caffeine begins to kick in, giving a double boost. Some find this method helpful, while others prefer to avoid caffeine because it could cause jitters or disrupt later sleep.

Tips if Trying It

- Do it at midday or early afternoon, not late.
- Keep the nap short. A long nap plus caffeine might cause more trouble at bedtime.

---

7. Naps and Overall Health

Short rests can have benefits beyond just giving a burst of energy. Some research suggests that controlled naps can reduce stress levels, improve memory, and aid in problem-solving. They may also help people who are learning new skills—when the brain gets a brief rest, it can better store and process new information.

However, relying on naps because of chronic poor nighttime rest is not the best long-term fix. If you use naps only to cope with not sleeping enough at night, it might be wise to address the root issue: poor sleep habits, stress, or a possible sleep disorder. A nap should be a supplement, not a replacement for solid nightly sleep.

8. Naps for Different Age Groups

8.1 Children

Young kids often nap during the day as part of normal development. Toddlers might nap once or twice a day. As they grow older, they gradually drop naps. By the time children reach school age, many no longer need a daily nap, though there are exceptions.

8.2 Teens

Teens require more sleep overall (often 8–10 hours). Because of early school times and late-night activities, many teens do not get enough rest at night, so they might feel the urge to nap after school. A short nap can help them study better, but a long late-afternoon nap might push bedtime even later, creating a cycle of late nights and groggy mornings.

8.3 Adults

Working adults might nap on weekends or try to squeeze in a lunch-break nap if work conditions allow. Some workplaces even have nap pods or quiet rooms now. For most adults, a brief midday rest can improve mood and alertness without too much risk of harming nighttime rest—provided it is not too late or too long.

8.4 Older Adults

Older people might wake earlier or have segmented rest at night. Napping can help make up for lost sleep. However, taking long naps close to the evening might lead to more difficulties at bedtime. Short midday naps can be beneficial if nighttime rest is often interrupted.

---

9. Cultural Differences in Napping

Some countries have a tradition of a midday rest or break, often in places with very warm climates. People may take a break after lunch, which can be used for a nap or just quiet time. This can shift their day so that bedtime is later. In other cultures, napping might be seen as something only for the very young, the old, or the ill. But modern science often shows that short rests can help almost anyone if used correctly.

10. Potential Downsides of Napping

1. **Interrupted Nighttime Rest**: The main risk is that a nap can reduce "sleep pressure," making it harder to fall asleep at night.
2. **Grogginess**: Waking from a deep stage can leave you feeling more tired than before if the nap is not timed well.
3. **Possible Social Stigma**: In workplaces or social settings where naps are not common, you might face criticism for lying down midday.
4. **Dependence**: If you rely heavily on naps to fix consistent lack of sleep, you might never address the real reasons you are not sleeping at night.

11. Sign You Might Be Napping for the Wrong Reasons

- You nap almost every day because you are exhausted, not just once in a while for a pick-me-up.
- You need long, 2–3 hour naps to feel "okay."
- You struggle with insomnia or frequent awakenings at night.
- You wake up from naps feeling worse than before.

In these cases, it may be time to look at your nighttime routine, environment, and overall health. A sleep disorder could be part of the problem. Or you might be pushing your body's schedule too hard.

12. Using Short Rests for Shift Workers

People who work night or rotating shifts often cannot stick to a typical sleep schedule. Naps become more essential to fill in gaps. A well-timed nap before a night shift, for example, can help reduce fatigue on the job. A brief rest after coming home might also help you feel better, but it is important not to push your main "core sleep" too close to your next shift. Creating a schedule that includes a core rest plus a planned nap can support better alertness.

13. If You Cannot Nap

Not everyone can sleep easily during the day, even when tired. Some people find daytime rest impossible because their bodies are very set to nighttime sleep. Others cannot relax enough due to work demands or lack of a quiet space. If you cannot nap, consider alternative ways to recharge:

- **Relaxing Break**: Spend 10-15 minutes with eyes closed in a quiet place, even if not fully asleep.
- **Gentle Stretching**: This can reduce muscle tension and perk you up slightly.
- **Fresh Air**: A quick walk outdoors can raise alertness.

These options may not replace sleep, but they can help you get through a slump if a nap is not an option.

14. Nap Environment

Just like nighttime sleep, environment matters for naps:

- **Darkness**: A dark room can help signal the mind to rest quickly. If you are at work, an eye mask might help.
- **Quiet**: Earplugs or noise-canceling headphones can block out distractions.
- **Comfortable Temperature**: Being too hot or too cold can ruin a nap.
- **Safe Spot**: If you are in an office or public place, choose somewhere you feel secure enough to relax.

15. Preparing for a Nap

- **Set an Alarm**: Decide on the nap length, then set an alarm so you do not overshoot.
- **Allow Transition Time**: After you wake up, give yourself a few minutes to fully come back to alertness before jumping back into complex tasks.
- **Stay Hydrated**: Sometimes a short rest plus a drink of water can do wonders. If you are dehydrated, you might feel more sluggish.

16. Napping and Mental Clarity

Studies show that short rests can improve mental clarity, reaction time, and even creativity for a few hours afterward. This can be very helpful for tasks that require focus or quick responses. In some jobs, like driving or operating machinery, a short rest break might reduce accidents caused by drowsiness.

---

17. Handling Nap-Related Guilt or Stigma

In cultures or environments where napping is seen as lazy, you might feel guilty. Yet, if you are consistently short on rest and a 20-minute rest helps you do better work or maintain a better mood, it could be a useful tool. If feasible, you might speak with a boss or coworkers about it, explaining that short breaks can boost performance. At home, you can set a house rule about quiet time, or coordinate with family so that your quick rest does not seem antisocial.

---

18. Travel and Jet Lag

When traveling across time zones, naps can either help or hinder. A short nap after arriving might help you get through the day if you are extremely tired, but a long daytime rest can stop you from adjusting to local nights. Balance is key. Aim for a controlled short rest and then push yourself to stay awake until local bedtime. Over a few days, your body may adapt faster.

---

19. Testing Your Nap Length

Because personal responses vary, a practical method is to test different lengths:

1. **Week 1**: Try 15–20-minute naps around 1:00 pm. Notice how you feel after waking and at bedtime.
2. **Week 2**: Test a 30–40-minute nap if you need more rest. Compare.
3. **Week 3**: If you still feel tired, try a 60-minute nap, but watch if bedtime becomes an issue.

Keep notes on how easy or hard it is to fall asleep that night, how you feel upon waking from the nap, and whether you experience grogginess or a second wind.

20. Final Thoughts on Napping

Naps can be a double-edged sword. Done at the right time and length, they can boost energy and mood. Done too late or too long, they might disrupt nighttime rest and lead to sluggishness. Whether you include naps in your daily routine depends on your lifestyle, work schedule, and how well you generally sleep at night.

Key Points

1. **Nap Length Matters**: 10-20 minutes is great for a quick reset. 30-60 minutes might provide more rest but can lead to grogginess. 90 minutes or more risks messing with nighttime sleep.
2. **Time of Day**: Early to mid-afternoon is usually best if you do not want bedtime delays.
3. **Environment**: A quiet, safe, and comfortable spot helps you fall asleep faster and wake feeling better.
4. **Listen to Your Body**: If naps consistently make you feel worse or wreck your sleep at night, they may not be right for you.
5. **Address Underlying Issues**: If you are always exhausted and feel you need daily naps, look into why your nighttime rest is not sufficient.

In the next chapters, we will continue examining different angles of rest, such as shifting how you think about sleep, how rest can differ by age, and the kinds of tools or gadgets people use to aid rest. Understanding how each piece fits together can help you build a daily life plan where you feel more alert during the day and more at peace during the night.

Chapter 15: Changing Your Thinking About Sleep

In earlier chapters, we explored many topics that affect your rest—like routines, stress, and bedroom conditions. Now, we will focus on the role your mind plays in helping or hurting your rest. Beliefs, thoughts, and worries can shape how quickly you fall asleep, whether you stay asleep, and how refreshed you feel in the morning. In this chapter, we will look at common thinking patterns that can make rest difficult, as well as ways to adjust those patterns. We will also discuss step-by-step methods you can try if you find your mind racing at night. By learning to see rest as a supportive, natural process, you can remove many of the mental roadblocks that keep you from drifting off easily.

1. The Influence of Thoughts on Sleep

The Power of the Mind
Your thoughts can either help you relax or keep you tense. If you climb into bed thinking, "I will never fall asleep," you might trigger stress signals in your body. The more stressed you feel, the harder it is to rest. This cycle can become so strong that even if you are physically tired, your mind will not settle.

The Mind-Body Link
When you are relaxed, your muscles loosen, heart rate goes down, and breathing becomes steady. If your mind starts to fill with worries or negative beliefs, your body shifts back to a more alert state. A calm mind encourages a calm body, and a calm body helps the mind let go of extra thoughts.

2. Common Negative Beliefs About Sleep

Many people hold beliefs that make rest seem difficult or even scary. Here are some examples:

1. **"I must get 8 hours of sleep or tomorrow will be ruined."**
    - This belief sets a strict rule that can create panic if you are not asleep on time. Some nights, 7 hours might be enough. Other nights, you might need a bit more. Being flexible can ease pressure.

2. **"Everyone else sleeps perfectly, but I cannot."**
   - In reality, many people struggle at times. Thinking that you are the only one with a problem can add shame or frustration. Understanding you are not alone can reduce stress.
3. **"If I wake up at night, it means something is wrong."**
   - Brief awakenings can be normal. Believing that they signal a serious issue can lead to overreaction. Waking up does not always mean bad rest, especially if you fall back asleep quickly.
4. **"Lying in bed with my mind racing means I am doomed to be tired tomorrow."**
   - A tense body and busy mind can stop rest, but it does not have to remain that way all night. You can learn ways to calm the mind and still get enough sleep.
5. **"I have tried everything, and nothing works."**
   - Many people try a few basic tips. However, deeper changes to thoughts, environment, and habits might take time. Also, new methods need consistent practice.

---

3. The Role of Worry in Keeping You Awake

Thinking Errors
When you worry in bed, you might fall into "what if" thinking, imagining worst-case scenarios for tomorrow. Thoughts like, "What if I fail that meeting because I am tired?" or "What if I get sick from lack of rest?" can fill your mind with fear, raising stress hormones.

Cycle of Anxiety
The more you worry, the more awake you feel. And the more awake you feel, the more you believe you cannot rest. This loop can repeat each night if not broken. You might end up dreading bedtime, which adds another layer of stress.

Worry Versus Planning
Worry often feels like planning, but it is usually repetitive and negative. Planning is more practical—deciding steps to solve a problem. If you catch yourself circling the same worries at bedtime, you can tell yourself, "I will handle these thoughts tomorrow when I can do something about them."

4. Shifting Your Thoughts

From Negative to Balanced
You do not have to force yourself into overly positive thinking. Instead, aim for balanced thoughts. For example, replace "I will never sleep tonight" with "I might have trouble drifting off, but I can use calm methods, and even lying quietly has some rest benefits." This new thought does not deny your struggle but also opens a path to gentle hope.

Building Confidence
Celebrate small successes. If you fall asleep 10 minutes faster than usual, recognize that as progress. Over time, you can reshape your mindset from "I always struggle" to "I am learning ways to rest better."

Question Old Beliefs
Ask yourself if a belief is 100% accurate. For instance, if you often say, "I cannot function on less than 8 hours," think about times you got 7 hours and still had a decent day. This does not mean you want less rest all the time, but it shows your body might adapt better than you think.

---

5. Dealing with Performance Pressure

The "Big Event" Problem
If you have an important test, job interview, or appointment the next day, you might feel intense pressure to sleep well. Ironically, that pressure can keep you awake. One rough night, however, does not always ruin the next day. Sometimes adrenaline and excitement help you manage even if your rest was not perfect.

Practical Steps

- **Plan Ahead**: If you know a big day is coming, try to keep a good routine for several nights before.
- **Relaxation**: Use deep breathing or muscle-release methods to reduce the tension caused by performance pressure.
- **Focus on Calm, Not on Sleeping**: Instead of thinking, "I must fall asleep now," think, "Let me stay calm and let rest come when it is ready."

6. Cognitive Methods for Better Rest

One formal approach to changing your thoughts about sleep is often called cognitive methods for rest. This involves noticing negative thoughts, challenging them, and replacing them with more balanced statements. It also includes some behaviors that train your mind and body to link bed with rest rather than worry.

6.1 Writing Down Concerns

Some people find that listing worries before bed frees the mind. You can schedule 10 minutes earlier in the evening to write down any tasks or problems. Then, if the worries come up later, remind yourself that you have them noted and can address them tomorrow. This can break the habit of mentally circling around the same concerns in bed.

6.2 Sleep Diary

A diary can help you see patterns. Write down:

- Time you went to bed
- Roughly how long it took to fall asleep
- Any awakenings or final wake-up time
- How rested you felt the next day

Over weeks, you might see that you are actually getting more rest than you thought, or that certain days you worry less and drift off faster.

6.3 Bed for Sleep Only

Avoid doing stressful activities (like work or heated talks) in bed. If you do many wakeful things in bed—like scrolling your phone, reading intense news—your mind starts connecting bed with staying alert. The goal is for your mind to link bed with calm and rest.

---

7. Breaking the Fear of Sleeplessness

Acceptance Approach
Trying to force yourself to sleep often backfires. Instead, an acceptance

approach suggests you let go of the battle. You might say, "Even if I lie awake, that is okay. I am still giving my body a chance to rest." Paradoxically, removing the strict demand for sleep can make drifting off easier.

Gentle Distraction
When your mind will not stop, a mild distraction can help. Some people use a mental exercise like counting backward from 100 by 3s. Others picture a calm scene in detail—like a quiet lake, noticing the soft water or gentle breeze. This distracts the brain from worries without exciting it.

---

8. Handling Middle-of-the-Night Wake-Ups

Avoid Clock-Watching
Staring at the clock and calculating how many hours are left can increase worry. Turn the clock away or use a cover. If you do wake up, try to remain calm. Notice if you feel physically tense—relax your muscles. If after 15-20 minutes you remain wide awake, get up and do something quiet in low light, like reading a calm book (nothing too exciting or stressful), then return to bed when you feel a bit sleepy again.

Positive Self-Talk
Rather than thinking, "Great, I am awake again, and this ruins my night," say, "I woke up, but I can still get enough rest. Let me stay relaxed and see what happens." This mind shift can keep stress levels low, allowing rest to return.

---

9. Realistic Sleep Expectations

Fluctuations Are Normal
No one sleeps exactly the same amount every single night. Some nights are shorter, some are longer, and that is normal. The body has a way of self-correcting over days or weeks if you have slight ups and downs.

Aim for Quality Over Quantity
Seven hours of high-quality rest can be more refreshing than nine hours of tossing and turning. Focus on how you feel rather than just the clock number. If

you are still feeling tired daily despite enough hours in bed, it could be that stress, environment, or a sleep disorder is interfering with quality.

Extra Sleep Is Not Always Better
Many people think if they are tired, they need to stay in bed longer. But lying in bed for too long—especially if awake—can actually worsen your sleep patterns. Sticking to a consistent wake-up time and focusing on better rest habits might be more effective than forcing extra hours.

---

10. Using Visualization

Visualization is the practice of creating calming pictures in your mind. Some find it easier to do with the help of a quiet audio guide, while others can do it alone. Examples include imagining a gentle waterfall or a peaceful forest walk, paying attention to soft details like the color of leaves or the sound of water. The point is not to have vivid daydreams that excite you, but to soothe the mind so it is not dwelling on stress or negative beliefs.

---

11. Self-Compassion When Struggling with Sleep

Being Kind to Yourself
If you have had trouble for months or years, it is easy to become harsh or blame yourself. But negative self-talk can make rest problems worse. Tell yourself you are learning, not failing. Recognize the effort you are making to improve your nights.

Comparisons to Others
Resist the urge to compare your rest to that of a friend or family member who claims they never have trouble. Every person's body and mind differ. Focusing on what you can control in your own situation is more productive than feeling bad about not matching someone else.

12. Tackling the "All or Nothing" Mindset

Some people see their sleep as a total success or total failure. If they wake up once, they feel it is all ruined. But rest can have many parts. You might doze off easily, then wake briefly, and still get enough good rest. Breaking free from an "all or nothing" mindset can reduce frustration. Realize that partial success—like fewer awakenings or quicker return to sleep—is still progress.

---

13. Looking at the Big Picture

Beyond Tonight
If you focus too much on each individual night, you might overlook broader patterns. A week or month approach can help. Maybe you had a few bad nights but overall improved compared to last month. This viewpoint encourages patience and keeps you from overreacting to a single poor night.

Lifestyle Factors
Remember that thoughts about rest are only part of the picture. Nutrition, exercise, environment, light exposure, and stress also contribute. Feeling hopeless about your nights might shift if you notice that daily walks or reducing caffeine actually help you rest better, proving that improvement is possible.

---

14. When to Seek Extra Help

Sometimes self-help approaches are not enough. If worry, sad moods, or emotional issues are causing major rest problems, a counselor or psychologist may offer specialized tools. They can teach structured methods to change unhelpful thoughts, manage worries, and shape healthy rest patterns. If you suspect a medical cause, like sleep apnea or other conditions, a doctor's evaluation is important.

15. Setting Gradual Goals

Short-Term Goals

- Aim to reduce the time spent worrying in bed by 10 minutes this week.
- Use one calming exercise, like slow breathing, each night before bed.

Long-Term Goals

- Build a more positive attitude toward bed, seeing it as a place of rest rather than stress.
- Maintain a stable routine for at least a month, noticing if your overall mood and energy improve.

---

16. Staying Motivated

Track Your Wins
Keep a small journal of positive changes. Maybe you fell asleep in 30 minutes instead of 60, or you only woke up once instead of three times. Write that down, so on tough nights, you can look back and see the progress.

Reward Yourself
When you hit a milestone (like sticking to a bedtime routine for two weeks), allow yourself a small treat or a relaxing activity. Positive reinforcement can help you continue building better habits.

---

17. Overcoming Setbacks

Expect Ups and Downs
Improving thoughts about rest is not always a straight line. You might have a good stretch, then experience stress from work or family, and revert to old patterns. Recognize this is normal. The key is returning to your constructive habits.

Do Not Catastrophize
If you have a few bad nights in a row, do not jump to "I am back to zero

progress." Instead, see them as a temporary challenge. Review what might have changed—more stress, less exercise, or big life events. Adjust as needed and remind yourself you have tools that worked before.

18. Additional Methods for Calming the Mind

1. **Hand Relaxation**: Lie in bed and slowly open and close your hands, focusing on the sensation. This can ground your mind in the present.
2. **Writing Gratitudes**: Some people find that listing a few good things from the day lifts mood and softens negative thought loops.
3. **Soundscapes**: Listening to soft nature sounds or repetitive gentle music can be a mental anchor, lulling you away from daily worries.

19. Integrating a Balanced View of Sleep

The goal is not to turn sleep into a source of stress, but to see it as a natural process the body is ready to do. Your job is mainly to create the conditions—physically and mentally—that allow it to happen. By adjusting your thinking and adopting calm strategies, you help the body return to its normal rhythms.

20. Putting It All Together

Changing how you think about sleep is a valuable step for overcoming long-term struggles. It involves shifting from negative, rigid beliefs to more balanced and understanding views, reducing worry, and learning helpful mental tools. You do not have to become a perfect thinker overnight. Even small mental shifts can reduce the stress that fuels restless nights.

Key Points

1. **Recognize Unhelpful Thoughts**: Notice and label thoughts that worsen tension, and practice forming balanced alternatives.

2. **Use Written Exercises**: A worry list or diary can free your mind from circling the same thoughts.
3. **Focus on Calm Instead of Forcing Sleep**: Gentle acceptance often works better than pressuring yourself to drop off.
4. **Set Realistic Goals**: Aiming to be "perfect" can add pressure. Seek gradual progress.
5. **Seek Support If Needed**: A mental health professional can offer deeper skills for changing thought patterns.

In the next chapter, we will look at how rest can vary across different stages of life, from infancy to older adulthood. Each phase brings unique challenges and solutions. By understanding these changes, you can support your own rest or help loved ones get the rest they need, no matter their age or stage.

Chapter 16: Sleep Across Different Ages

Age influences almost every aspect of rest. Infants need far more hours than adults, teenagers have shifting patterns, and older adults can face unique challenges with waking up early or having lighter sleep. In this chapter, we will discuss rest requirements and common issues faced at each life stage. We will also offer simple methods to support better rest for babies, children, teens, adults, and seniors. Whether you have young kids in the house or you are caring for an older family member, understanding these age-related differences can help everyone sleep better.

1. Infants and Toddlers

1.1 Newborns

Sleep Duration
Newborns can sleep 14 to 17 hours a day, often in short bursts of 2-4 hours around the clock. Their internal clocks are not yet developed, so day and night do not mean much to them.

Feeding and Sleep
Newborns wake frequently to eat. As they grow, these feeds spread out, and they gradually stay awake longer between naps. Some parents feel stressed by the constant cycle of feeding and sleeping.

Tips

- **Safe Environment**: Always follow safety guidelines for the baby's bed. Avoid loose blankets or objects in the crib.
- **Daytime Light**: Expose the baby to soft daylight during the day to start shaping the internal clock.
- **Nighttime Quiet**: Keep lights dim and noise low at night, so the baby starts to sense it is rest time.

1.2 Older Babies (3–12 Months)

Developing Patterns
At around 3 months or older, babies start to have longer nighttime stretches and more predictable nap times. They might sleep 12-15 hours total, including naps.

Challenges

- **Teething**: Pain can disrupt rest.
- **Separation Worries**: Some babies cry when parents are not nearby.
- **Routine Changes**: Travel or illness can temporarily throw off schedules.

Tips

- **Consistent Bedtime Routine**: A short pattern of a bath, a lullaby, or gentle rocking can signal bedtime.
- **Soothing Items**: Some babies like a special blanket (safe and sized properly) or a soft night light.
- **Avoid Overstimulation Before Bed**: Loud play or bright screens can keep them wired.

1.3 Toddlers (1–3 Years)

Energy and Curiosity
Toddlers are exploring the world. They usually need around 12-14 hours of rest, often with one or two daytime naps, which might drop to one nap as they approach age 3.

Bedtime Battles
Toddlers might resist bedtime because they want to keep playing or they test limits. Consistent rules and clear routines help them settle down.

Tips

- **Wind-Down Time**: Calm activities, like reading a simple book, are better than rowdy games before bed.
- **Offer Choices**: Let them pick which pajamas to wear or which stuffed animal to have—small choices can ease power struggles.
- **Stay Consistent**: Even if they protest, maintain a regular bedtime.

2. Preschoolers and School-Age Children

2.1 Preschoolers (3–5 Years)

Imagination and Fears

Preschoolers might have vivid imaginations. Nightmares or fear of the dark can begin. They need about 10-13 hours total, often including an afternoon nap, though some drop napping by 5 years old.

Tips

- **Night Light**: A small, dim light can ease fear of darkness.
- **Reassuring Tone**: Let them know they are safe. Briefly check on them if they call out, but avoid turning bedtime into a big game or a long interaction.
- **Limit Screen Use**: Bright cartoons or tablet games close to bedtime can make them wired.

2.2 School-Age Children (6–12 Years)

Increased Responsibilities

Children at this age have homework, activities, and social events. Sleep often drops to 9-12 hours. Busy schedules might lead them to go to bed too late.

Tips

- **Regular Schedule**: Even though they have more going on, keep a consistent bedtime.
- **Quiet Hour**: Encourage them to do calmer activities before bed, like reading or drawing, instead of exciting games.
- **Technology Limits**: Try to keep TVs, tablets, or phones out of their bedroom if possible.

---

3. Teenagers (13–19 Years)

3.1 Biological Shifts

Teens often feel sleepy later at night because their bodies release certain hormones on a delayed schedule. They might naturally want to go to bed at 11 pm or midnight and sleep until 8 or 9 am. But school start times often clash with this, leading many teens to be short on rest.

3.2 Rest Needs

Most teens need 8–10 hours. But with early school days, many only get 6–7. This shortfall can cause mood swings, trouble focusing, and lower academic performance.

3.3 Social Demands

Teens may stay up texting friends or scrolling social media. Light from screens and the mental stimulation can push bedtime later. Weekend "catch-up" sleeping can worsen the mismatch by shifting their body clock even more.

3.4 Tips

- **Consistent Sleep-Wake Schedule**: Encourage them to keep a regular bedtime and wake-up time, even on weekends (with a bit of flexibility).
- **Screen Curfew**: Aim to stop phone or device use at least 30–60 minutes before bed.
- **Nap Carefully**: A short after-school nap might help if they are extremely tired, but keep it brief and before late afternoon.
- **Discuss Priorities**: Help them see that proper rest can improve mood, grades, and sports performance.

---

4. Young Adults (20–39 Years)

4.1 Busy Lifestyles

College, jobs, social events, and possibly starting a family—young adults have packed schedules. They might stay up late to finish work or go out. Rest can become an afterthought, leading to chronic tiredness.

4.2 Rest Requirements

Most adults in this age range do well with 7–9 hours. Some might manage on 6 if the quality is very good, but consistent lack of rest eventually shows in reduced focus or health problems.

4.3 Tips

- **Set Boundaries**: With so many demands, it is vital to guard bedtime from constant interruptions.
- **Watch Caffeine and Alcohol**: Both can reduce quality if consumed too late.
- **Balance Social Life**: Occasional late nights might be fine, but if it becomes a habit, it can seriously affect health.
- **Nap Wisely**: A short midday nap can help if nighttime rest is lacking, but avoid late or long naps.

---

5. Middle Adulthood (40–59 Years)

5.1 Hormonal Changes

Some adults experience shifts in hormone levels, especially women approaching menopause. Hot flashes or night sweats can interrupt rest. Men may see changes in energy or new health concerns that affect their nights.

5.2 Work and Family Stress

Jobs might be at a peak of responsibility, and caring for children or older parents can add stress and reduce time for proper rest. Stress hormones can remain high, making it tough to wind down.

5.3 Tips

- **Manage Stress**: Use methods like gentle exercise, calming hobbies, or short breaks to reduce tension.
- **Bedroom Adjustments**: Cooling the room or using light bedding can help with hot flashes or general overheating.
- **Check Health Issues**: High blood pressure, joint pains, or other conditions might need treatment to protect your rest.
- **Stay Active**: Regular physical activity aids mood and can help regulate rest cycles, as long as it is not too close to bedtime.

6. Older Adulthood (60+ Years)

6.1 Changes in Sleep Patterns

Seniors might fall asleep earlier in the evening and wake up very early in the morning. They could also have lighter, more fragmented rest, leading to multiple awakenings at night. Despite this, they often still need around 7-8 hours, though it can be split differently.

6.2 Common Issues

- **Frequent Bathroom Trips**: Bladder changes or medications can cause night awakenings.
- **Health Conditions**: Aches, arthritis, or illnesses can cause discomfort.
- **Medication Side Effects**: Some drugs can cause drowsiness or insomnia.

6.3 Tips

- **Consistent Routines**: Having a set bedtime and wake-up time helps stabilize the body clock.
- **Daytime Light Exposure**: Getting sunlight early in the day can reinforce wakefulness in the morning and sleepiness at night.
- **Address Pain**: If pain disrupts rest, talk to a health professional about timing of meds or other pain relief methods.
- **Mindful Naps**: A short nap might refresh, but a long or late one can reduce nighttime rest.

---

7. Special Concerns

7.1 Shift Workers

Regardless of age, shift workers must often rest during the day and stay awake at night. This goes against the natural circadian rhythm. Using blackout curtains, limiting morning light after a night shift, and sticking to a consistent sleep schedule can help. Age can make these challenges tougher, but the same core tips apply.

7.2 People with Chronic Conditions

Some health conditions—like diabetes, heart disease, or chronic pain—can appear at different ages and disrupt rest. Working closely with medical professionals to manage symptoms, adopting good rest habits, and adjusting environment can help you rest better, no matter your age.

---

8. Family Considerations and Multiple Age Groups

Many households have family members at different life stages. A baby might cry at night, waking a parent who has an early job. A teen might stay up late playing games, disturbing younger siblings. Balancing these needs can be tough.

Ideas

- **Quiet Hours**: Set times when noise is kept low.
- **Separate Spaces**: If possible, give a restless teen a room away from a baby's nursery.
- **Shared Routines**: Eating dinner together at a reasonable time and turning off devices an hour before bed can help the entire family wind down.

---

9. Recognizing Sleep Needs as You Age

Self-Awareness
Pay attention to how your rest changes. Maybe you need to go to bed a bit earlier in your 50s than you did in your 30s. Or maybe you need a 10-minute wind-down stretch in your 70s to ease stiff joints before lying down. Adjust gradually and do not force yourself into the exact same pattern you had at a younger age.

Avoid Self-Judgment
Some older adults think it is lazy to sleep longer, or they worry something is wrong because they wake up earlier. Checking with a doctor is wise if you suspect real problems, but mild shifts in pattern are often natural.

---

10. Life Events That Can Affect Sleep

1. **Pregnancy**: In addition to physical changes, hormone shifts can cause increased tiredness and nighttime bathroom breaks. As pregnancy advances, finding a comfortable position may require pillows for support.
2. **Menopause**: Hot flashes, mood swings, and other changes can disrupt rest. It helps to keep the room cool, avoid spicy foods close to bedtime, and explore methods to reduce discomfort.
3. **Major Stress or Loss**: Any serious life event can affect rest at any age. Approaches like counseling, stress management, or a support group can be helpful.

---

11. Adapting Habits for Each Stage

While the basics—like a good environment, consistent bedtime, and avoiding late-night stimulants—are important for everyone, the exact approach can vary by age. For instance:

- **Babies**: They thrive on a predictable routine, but they still wake up often for feeding.
- **Teens**: Might need guidance to limit devices and shift bedtime a bit earlier.
- **Adults**: Might need to schedule short breaks or reduce late caffeine if they see signs of burnout.
- **Seniors**: Could benefit from mild evening exercise or stretching to reduce aches.

---

12. Communication Within the Household

If you are a parent, talking to kids about why rest matters can help them accept bedtime rules. Teens might not always listen, but explaining how it impacts mood and performance can slowly influence them. Older adults living with you might have different routines, so coordinating schedules can prevent clashes—for example, if a grandparent wakes at 5 am and starts making noise while others are sleeping.

13. Technology and Age

Children may be drawn to tablets or phones at night. Teens practically live on their smartphones. Young adults juggle laptops for work. Middle-aged folks might watch late-night news. Seniors might fall asleep with the TV on. Each age group can have a technology habit that disrupts rest. Setting device-free times or areas can help everyone, though older family members might be used to falling asleep with the TV on. If that is the case, suggest a timer that shuts it off after a certain period.

14. Changing Sleep Patterns in Older Adults: Myths vs. Realities

Myth: Older adults need far less rest.
Reality: They still need a similar amount, though how it is divided might shift.

Myth: Waking at night means there is a serious problem.
Reality: Waking briefly can be normal if one can fall back asleep.

Myth: Afternoon dozing is always harmful.
Reality: A short rest can be refreshing, but hours-long naps can reduce nighttime rest quality.

15. Different Bed Times for Couples

It is not unusual for spouses or partners of different ages (or with different work hours) to have separate sleep-wake times. One might be an "early bird," the other a "night owl." Communication and compromise can help so that one person's schedule does not disrupt the other's. Some couples find sleeping in slightly separate routines or separate rooms solves snoring or schedule conflicts, and that is okay if it works for them.

16. Transition Phases and Sleep

College/Leaving Home
Young people might go from a household with a set bedtime to a dorm with no rules. This can lead to late nights and irregular patterns. Encouraging self-awareness about rest can reduce harmful habits.

Retirement
Suddenly not having to wake for work might tempt some to stay up late or sleep in. Setting a loose schedule can keep them feeling good. Overly irregular habits might lead to poor rest and less energy for daytime activities.

---

17. Teaching Children and Teens About Sleep

Simple Explanations
Kids can understand that rest is when the body and brain refuel, just like a phone charging. Teens can learn about how the internal clock shifts, so they see it is not just "laziness" but biology.

Modeling Good Habits
If parents are glued to screens late at night, children pick up that behavior. Showing them that you prioritize your own rest can make them more likely to respect bedtime rules.

---

18. Emotional Changes with Age and Sleep

A teen might have stress from school or friendships, while a middle-aged person might worry about finances, and an older adult might feel lonely or anxious about health. Each emotion can impact rest. Recognizing that different ages face different emotional pressures helps us show empathy. For instance, a child's fear of monsters is real to them, just like a teen's worry about an exam or an adult's worry about retirement funds. Each concern can lead to sleepless nights if not handled kindly.

19. Professional Guidance for Each Age

1. **Babies and Toddlers**: Pediatricians can give advice on feeding, bedtime routines, and dealing with frequent awakenings.
2. **Kids and Teens**: School counselors or doctors can help if they show signs of heavy tiredness, sadness, or ongoing difficulty with rest.
3. **Adults**: Seeing a doctor if you suspect issues like apnea or hormonal imbalances is important. A mental health specialist can help if stress or sadness is a factor.
4. **Seniors**: Geriatric specialists can address concerns like pain management, medication side effects, or conditions that disrupt rest (like restless legs or chronic conditions).

---

20. Bringing It All Together

Age affects how much rest we need and how we get it—whether in many short bursts as a baby, or earlier bedtimes as we age. Each life phase has unique problems and solutions. Yet, across all ages, the key remains: support healthy habits, keep a calm mindset, and address any physical or emotional barriers.

Key Points

1. **Babies**: Focus on safety and gentle routines.
2. **Children**: Maintain consistent bedtimes, limit screens, and address fears.
3. **Teens**: Understand their natural shift to later bedtimes, but encourage a stable schedule and limited late-night device use.
4. **Adults**: Balance work, family, and social life with enough rest. Watch stress and substance use.
5. **Older Adults**: Adapt to changing patterns, address health issues, and aim for a routine that fits new rhythms.

Knowing what is normal (and what is not) for each age can reduce worry and guide practical steps. In the next chapter, we will look at helpful tools and gadgets that people of different ages use to improve rest. From simple items like pillows and fans to more advanced apps and trackers, we will explore which ones might truly help—and how to use them wisely without adding more stress.

Chapter 17: Helpful Tools and Gadgets

You have already learned about the importance of creating the right environment, managing stress, adjusting nutrition, and more. Sometimes, however, a few well-chosen tools or devices can provide added support for your rest. Modern items range from simple and inexpensive to very high-tech. But not all gadgets live up to their promises. In this chapter, we will examine a range of options—mattresses, pillows, white noise machines, apps, and trackers, among others—and discuss how to choose them wisely. We will also touch on how to use them without letting them become a distraction.

1. Mattress Types and Considerations

Your bed is one of the most important "tools" you have. A supportive, comfortable mattress can make a major difference in how well you rest. There are several categories:

1. **Innerspring**: Traditional design with coils. Often provides a bouncy feel. Quality can vary widely.
2. **Memory Foam**: Molds to the body. Good for pressure relief, but some traps heat. Modern versions often have cooling features.
3. **Latex**: Responsive like foam but usually cooler. Can be natural or synthetic.
4. **Hybrid**: Mix of coils and foam or latex layers. Aims to blend support with comfort.
5. **Air Beds**: Chambers inflated to desired firmness. Some allow separate settings on each side.

Things to Note

- **Firmness Preference**: A side sleeper might need a softer top layer for shoulder and hip relief. A back sleeper often likes medium. A stomach sleeper may prefer something on the firmer side.
- **Motion Transfer**: If you share a bed, a mattress that minimizes motion transfer (often foam or hybrid) can keep one person's movement from disturbing the other.

- **Trial Period**: Some companies let you test a mattress for a few weeks or months. This can be helpful since quick store tests do not always show how you will feel after a full night.

---

2. Pillows and Special Support

Pillows are a second line of defense for alignment and comfort. An unsuitable pillow can lead to neck and shoulder discomfort. Consider these points:

1. **Loft (Height)**: Different sleeping positions require different pillow heights.
   - **Side Sleepers**: Usually need more loft to keep head in line with spine.
   - **Back Sleepers**: Often do well with medium loft.
   - **Stomach Sleepers**: Usually need thin or no pillow to prevent excess neck strain.
2. **Materials**:
   - **Memory Foam**: Provides contouring but can trap heat if not ventilated.
   - **Down or Feather**: Soft and adjustable, but can flatten over time; also not suitable for some allergies.
   - **Latex**: Firmer feel but good support.
   - **Buckwheat Hull**: Adjusts to head shape, good airflow, but might be noisy or heavy.
3. **Specialty Pillows**:
   - **Body Pillows**: Helpful for side sleepers who want to support arms and legs or reduce back twisting.
   - **Wedge Pillows**: Good for propping up the upper body, possibly easing acid reflux or snoring.
   - **Cervical Pillows**: Designed to maintain neck curvature. Might help with certain neck or spine issues.

---

3. White Noise and Soothing Sound Machines

Noise disrupts rest. However, a steady background sound—like gentle static or rain—can mask sudden changes in noise that might awaken you. That is where white noise or other "color" noise devices come in:

1. **White Noise Machines**: Emit a consistent, neutral sound.
2. **Pink Noise**: Similar to white noise but balanced to be gentler for some ears.
3. **Nature Sounds**: Devices or apps might offer rainfall, ocean waves, or forest sounds.
4. **Fan**: A simple electric fan can produce a steady hum, which some find soothing.

Things to Consider

- **Volume**: It should not be so loud that it damages hearing or becomes another distraction.
- **Sound Type**: Some prefer rain or ocean waves, others like the steady hush of white noise.
- **Loop Quality**: Some cheaper machines or apps have obvious loops or crackles that can bother sensitive ears.

---

4. Aromatherapy and Diffusers

Some people use mild scents to create a calmer mood. A diffuser that releases a light mist or a few drops of mild oil on a cotton ball can produce a gentle smell in the bedroom:

- **Options**: Mild scents from plants like certain mint varieties or certain flowers. Avoid very strong or sharp fragrances.
- **Safety**: If you share a bedroom, note that some people are sensitive to scents. Overdoing it can cause breathing irritation.
- **Quality**: Cheaper diffusers might leak or break easily. Look for ones that distribute scent evenly but not too powerfully.

(Reminder: We avoid certain fancy words. We'll just say "mild scents from plants like certain mint varieties or certain flowers." No mention of "essential oils" by brand name or the like. Keep it general.)

---

5. Phone Apps for Relaxation and Tracking

A huge range of apps claim to help with rest. They fall into several categories:

1. **Meditation or Calm Guidance**: Provide short audio sessions that guide you through breathing or simple mental exercises.
2. **Sound Apps**: Offer white noise, nature sounds, or soft music.
3. **Tracking Apps**: Use your phone's motion sensors or microphone to estimate rest patterns, snoring, or awakenings.

Potential Problems

- **Screen Light**: Staring at a bright screen can keep you alert. Use night modes or dim settings if you must look at the app.
- **Over-Tracking**: Some individuals become anxious about the data, obsessing over small changes in "sleep scores." This can lead to more stress.
- **Accuracy**: Consumer-level apps often provide rough estimates, not a perfect measure of your rest stages.

---

6. Wearable Trackers and Smartwatches

Wrist-worn devices can track movement, heart rate, and sometimes blood oxygen levels to guess how long and how deeply you rest. Some also offer features like silent alarms (vibration instead of sound) to wake you gently. These can give helpful clues if you suspect you are not sleeping as well as you think.

Points to Keep in Mind

- **Comfort**: Wearing a watch or band at night might bother some people.
- **Battery Life**: Some trackers need charging daily, which can conflict with wearing it at night.
- **Data Anxiety**: Similar to phone apps, constant monitoring may make some people worry too much.

7. Smart Lights and Dimmers

Light strongly affects the body clock. Smart bulbs and dimmers let you control brightness and color:

1. **Waking Up**: A lamp that gradually brightens in the morning can mimic dawn, potentially making it easier to wake.
2. **Winding Down**: Lights that dim and shift to warm hues in the evening can signal the body to get ready for rest.
3. **Automatic Schedules**: Some systems let you set times for lights to change, so you do not have to remember each night.

Concerns

- **Cost**: High-quality smart bulbs and hubs can be pricey.
- **Simplicity**: Some systems are complicated to set up. If it causes stress, it might not be worth it.

8. Specialized Alarm Clocks

Not everyone likes a harsh beep first thing in the morning. Some alternative alarm clocks:

1. **Sunrise Simulators**: Gradually increase light intensity, sometimes paired with soft sounds like gentle bird calls.
2. **Vibration Alarms**: A pad under the pillow or mattress vibrates to wake you silently. Good for heavy sleepers or shared bedrooms where you do not want to wake someone else.
3. **App Alarms**: Some apps claim to measure rest cycles and wake you at the lightest stage. This feature can be hit-or-miss, depending on the phone's sensors and your movement.

9. Earplugs and Eye Masks

Two very simple, affordable tools:

- **Earplugs**: Foam or silicone plugs can block out traffic, a partner's snoring, or other sounds. Quality varies, so you might need to try a few kinds to find the most comfortable ones.

- **Eye Masks**: Helpful if you do not have blackout curtains. Choose a mask that fits snugly but not too tight. Some are shaped to keep fabric away from your eyelashes, avoiding irritation.

These items are especially handy when traveling or if you have a roommate or family members who watch TV or make noise at night.

10. Fans, Air Purifiers, and Humidifiers

The temperature and air quality of your bedroom are also important:

- **Fans**: Provide both airflow and white noise.
- **Air Purifiers**: Filter dust or allergens, which might help if you wake up congested.
- **Humidifiers**: Add moisture to very dry air, reducing throat or nasal dryness. Conversely, if your room is too humid, a dehumidifier might help.

Safety and Maintenance

- Always clean devices to avoid mold or bacteria buildup, especially with humidifiers.
- Check filter replacements on air purifiers.

11. Gadgets for Snoring and Mild Sleep Issues

If a person has mild snoring that is not linked to a serious condition like sleep apnea, some tools might help:

1. **Nasal Strips**: Open nasal passages a bit, which can reduce snoring for some.
2. **Nasal Dilators**: Small devices placed in the nostrils to keep them open.
3. **Position Aids**: Some belts or pillow systems gently discourage back-sleeping if that worsens snoring.

Important: If snoring is very loud or includes gasping, it could be sleep apnea, which usually needs professional evaluation. Gadget fixes alone might not be enough.

12. Weighted Blankets

Weighted blankets contain pellets or beads that add extra weight, providing a feeling some find soothing. This can help with restlessness or mild worries at night. However, it is not for everyone:

- **Choose Proper Weight**: Usually 10% of your body weight is suggested, though personal preference varies.
- **Temperature**: Some find these blankets too hot. Now there are "cooling" weighted blankets with breathable fabrics.
- **Safety**: Not suitable for infants or very small children. Anyone with certain health issues should consult a doctor first.

13. Recliners and Adjustable Beds

Some people, particularly those with reflux or certain back issues, prefer partially upright positions:

- **Recliners**: A comfortable chair that tilts back can be where some older adults or those with breathing difficulties sleep better. But long-term, it might reduce normal bed use, which has other drawbacks.
- **Adjustable Frames**: Can lift the head or legs. This might help circulation, back pain, or reduce snoring by opening airways. These can be expensive, so weigh the cost against the benefits.

14. Blue Light Glasses and Screen Filters

People who use devices in the evening might look into:

- **Blue Light–Blocking Glasses**: Tinted lenses that claim to block some of the short-wavelength light that keeps the brain alert.
- **Screen Filter Apps**: Shift device color temperature to warmer tones. Many phones and computers have a built-in "night mode."

Possible Concerns

- **Effectiveness**: Studies show mixed results. They might help a bit, but the best solution is often reducing screen time before bed.
- **Over-Reliance**: Wearing special glasses while still scrolling late into the night may not solve the underlying issue of mental stimulation.

---

15. Travel-Specific Tools

When you travel, your normal environment is gone. You can bring certain compact gadgets:

1. **Travel White Noise Machine**: Small, battery-powered devices or apps on your phone.
2. **Portable Pillow**: Neck pillows for planes or small versions of your normal pillow if you dislike hotel pillows.
3. **Compact Eye Mask**: Block out unfamiliar lights.
4. **Earplugs**: Essential in planes, trains, or loud hotels.

---

16. Balancing Gadgets with Simplicity

It is easy to become overwhelmed by all the available gear. Some people fill their rooms with high-tech devices, but that can lead to too many stimuli. The goal is to use tools that solve specific problems, not to crowd your night routine with more tasks.

---

17. Trying New Tools Safely

1. **Read Reviews**: Look for honest feedback, not just the marketing claims.
2. **Check Return Policies**: Some items, especially bigger-ticket products like mattresses, can be returned if you find them unsatisfactory.
3. **Test One at a Time**: If you add too many new tools at once, you will not know which one actually helps or if they conflict with each other.

4. **Monitor Effects**: Use a simple diary or mental notes to see if your rest or mood improves after adopting a new gadget.

18. Avoiding Gadget-Related Anxiety

Some folks get anxious about device measurements or settings. For instance, a tracker that says "You slept poorly" can lead to feeling worried all day, even if you actually feel fine. If data becomes stressful, it might be better to step away from continuous tracking.

19. Practical Tips for Minimizing Distractions

- **Set Up Once**: Adjust alarms, lights, or white noise settings before you start your wind-down routine so you are not fiddling with apps at bedtime.
- **Use Offline Modes**: If you rely on a phone for white noise, switch the phone to airplane mode so notifications do not interrupt.
- **Keep Tech Out of Reach**: If you have trouble resisting phone checks, place it out of arm's reach.

20. Pulling It All Together

Tools and gadgets can be a great support for rest if chosen and used thoughtfully. Before investing in something new, identify the specific issue you want to address—noise, temperature, neck support, etc.—then pick a product designed to help. Start with simpler or less costly solutions (like earplugs, a different pillow, or a fan) before moving on to bigger or pricier gear (smart beds, advanced sleep trackers). Always remember that no tool will fix poor routines or high stress by itself. These devices work best as part of a broader plan that includes stable bedtime hours, a calm mindset, and a healthy environment.

Key Points

1. **Bed Basics First**: A good mattress and pillow are central.

2. **Environment Aids**: White noise machines, fans, or simple earplugs often solve noise issues.
3. **Tech Tools**: Apps, trackers, and smart devices can help but might add complexity or cause worry.
4. **Check Real Impact**: Use diaries or simple observation to see if a gadget truly helps.
5. **Stay Balanced**: Do not let gear overshadow core habits like a consistent bedtime or avoiding large amounts of caffeine late in the day.

In the next chapter, we will examine how to maintain good rest when you are away from home. Travel, overnight visits, and unfamiliar rooms can all disrupt rest patterns. By planning ahead and taking along a few essentials, you can support better rest no matter where you are.

Chapter 18: Sleeping Away From Home

Many of us spend most nights in our own bedrooms, where we can control light, noise, and temperature. But what happens when you travel for work, stay at a hotel, spend the night with friends or family, or go camping? Different settings can disrupt your routine, leading to sleepless nights. This chapter will focus on practical tips for handling rest challenges when you are away from your usual environment. We will look at hotels, guest rooms, and even outdoor settings, and discuss ways to keep a sense of calm and comfort no matter where you lay your head.

1. Hotel Stays: Dealing with Unknown Surroundings

1.1 Room Requests

When booking a hotel, there are a few options you can consider to increase your chances of a good night's rest:

- **Higher Floors**: Often quieter, as you avoid street noise.
- **Away from Elevators**: Rooms near elevator banks can be noisy with foot traffic.
- **Non-Smoking Floor**: If you are sensitive to smells.
- **Ask About Events**: Some hotels host weddings or parties. Request a quieter wing if you suspect noise.

1.2 The Hotel Bed

Hotel mattresses vary. If you know you prefer firm or soft, call in advance to see if they have multiple firmness levels or a topper. Bring your own small pillow if you often struggle with the hotel's stock pillows.

1.3 Minimizing Light and Noise

- **Curtains**: Many hotels use heavy blackout drapes. Make sure you close them properly so street lights or early sun does not slip in.
- **Door Gaps**: Hall light can creep under the door. A rolled towel can block it.

- **Earplugs or White Noise**: Useful if walls are thin or if there is loud air conditioning. Some phone apps can help, but remember to use an offline mode if you do not want late notifications.

1.4 Keeping Routine

Try to keep parts of your bedtime routine the same. If you always read for 15 minutes or do gentle stretches, do so in your hotel room. Familiar actions can signal your mind that it is time to rest, even if the bed is unfamiliar.

---

2. Staying with Friends or Family

2.1 Communication

If you are visiting someone else's home, talk about your rest preferences politely. Maybe you need the room to be cooler or want to avoid loud music late at night. Clear and kind communication can help them understand your needs.

2.2 Guest Rooms or Sofas

You might be on a couch, a futon, or an air mattress. Try to bring items that add comfort:

- **Your Own Pillowcase**: A small touch of familiarity.
- **Earplugs and Eye Mask**: In case the living room has lights or the family wakes up early for breakfast.
- **Folded Blanket for Support**: If the sofa cushions are thin, placing a folded blanket beneath you can add padding.

2.3 Household Schedules

Some homes stay up late with the TV on. Others wake early. Ask about typical routines so you can adapt. If kids or pets are around, they might roam in the early morning. Ask if you can keep a door closed or if there is a quieter spot.

---

3. Business Travel and Jet Lag

3.1 Time Zone Shifts

If you fly east or west across multiple zones, your internal clock might not match the local day-night cycle. This is known as jet lag. Symptoms include feeling sleepy at odd times, waking too early, or having trouble falling asleep when you want to.

Strategies

- **Gradual Shift**: A few days before traveling, try going to bed and waking slightly closer to the new zone's time.
- **Light Exposure**: Spend time in the sunlight soon after arriving to help reset your clock.
- **Short Naps**: If you are extremely tired, a 20–30-minute midday rest can help, but avoid long naps that push your bedtime too late.
- **Stay Hydrated**: Air travel can dehydrate you, worsening fatigue.

3.2 Business Demands

You might have late dinners with clients or early morning meetings. If possible, plan a buffer day to adjust before diving into tight schedules. Keep an eye on caffeine intake; it might help you stay alert in the afternoon but harm your rest that night.

---

4. Camping and Outdoor Adventures

Sleeping outdoors adds unique challenges like temperature swings, ground hardness, and wildlife noises:

- **Tent and Sleeping Bag**: Invest in a sleeping bag suited to the expected weather. The rating should match the overnight lows.
- **Sleeping Pad**: A foam or inflatable pad reduces pressure from the ground and insulates against cold.
- **Temperature Control**: Dress in layers. A hat can keep heat from escaping if nights are cold. In warm climates, choose a well-ventilated tent.
- **Noise and Wildlife**: Crickets or distant animals can be loud. Some enjoy it; others prefer earplugs.

5. Napping While Away

If you are on a long car trip or traveling by plane, napping can help. But plan carefully:

1. **Car Trips**: If you are a passenger, a neck pillow can support your head. If you are driving, never nap behind the wheel. Park in a safe place.
2. **Planes or Trains**: A travel pillow, eye mask, and possibly noise-canceling headphones can help you doze in an upright seat.
3. **Time of Day**: Keep it short and not too late. A 20-minute nap might refresh you without ruining your nighttime rest.

6. Maintaining Routine on the Road

We talked about consistency in earlier chapters, and it remains key when away:

- **Meal Times**: Try not to shift meal times too much. Large late-night dinners on trips might keep you awake.
- **Exercise**: If you usually move regularly, try a short walk or simple stretches in your hotel room.
- **Lights Out**: Stick as close as possible to your usual bedtime or at least a window near that time.

7. Dealing with Different Beds

From a hotel mattress to a relative's couch, you may not have the comfort of home. A few adjustments can help:

- **Blanket or Towel**: Add softness under your hips or shoulders if you are a side sleeper.
- **Pillow Workarounds**: If the pillow is too high, use a rolled towel as a smaller pillow. If it is too flat, fold a sweater and place it under the pillow.
- **Position**: If a bed sags in the middle, try placing pillows to support your lower back.

8. Temperature and Climate Changes

Traveling often means going to places with different climates:

1. **Hot, Humid Areas**: Seek air conditioning or a fan. Stay hydrated. Shower or bathe to cool down before bed.
2. **Cold Places**: Layers of blankets, warm socks, maybe a hot water bottle at your feet.
3. **Altitude**: High altitude can cause breathing changes and poor rest until you adapt.

9. Hotel Noise from Hallways or Neighbors

Some hotels have thin walls:

- **Call the Front Desk**: If neighbors are too loud late at night, politely ask the front desk to help with a noise complaint.
- **Request a Room Change**: If you are near a loud ice machine or rowdy guests, it might be worth moving.
- **White Noise Apps**: Again, a phone or small device can fill the silence with a steady hum, masking sudden sounds.

10. Overcoming Anxiety About Sleeping Elsewhere

It is common to feel uneasy in a new place. The bed is different, you may not feel as safe, or you might worry about oversleeping if you have an early meeting:

- **Familiar Items**: Something simple like your pillowcase or a comfy T-shirt as pajamas can provide a sense of home.
- **Relaxation Routines**: Practice the same gentle breathing or mental exercises you do at home.
- **Night Light**: If you are anxious in new spaces, a small light can help you see where you are if you wake suddenly.

11. Handling Late Nights with Others

If you are visiting family or friends who like to stay up chatting, you might need to excuse yourself when it is your normal bedtime:

- **Polite Exit**: Thank them for the evening, mention an early morning or a need to rest, and head to your sleeping area.
- **Set Boundaries**: If you do not want to watch late-night shows, let them know kindly. You are a guest, but you also need to protect your well-being.

12. When Traveling with Kids

Children might already have their own routines. Traveling can throw them off:

1. **Keep Routines Where Possible**: Bring their favorite bedtime book or stuffed toy.
2. **Explain Changes**: If bedtime might be later, let them know in advance, but try to keep it only slightly different.
3. **Calming Activities**: If you are stuck in a hotel, use a corner of the room for quiet reading or coloring before bed.
4. **Address Fears**: Being in a strange place can lead to extra worries about monsters or noises. Reassure them or use a small night light.

13. Handling Late Dinners or Social Events

If you are staying with relatives or friends who eat dinner at 9 pm but you usually eat at 6 pm, this can affect rest:

- **Light Snacks**: If a meal is much later, have a small bite at your normal dinner time so you are not starving, but save enough appetite to join them.
- **Limit Heavy Foods**: If you do eat a big meal late, allow some digestion time before lying down. Maybe suggest a short walk together afterward.

14. Tech Use Away from Home

When away, you might rely on your phone or tablet more for navigation, communication, or entertainment:

- **Screen Curfew**: Even while traveling, try to limit bright screens right before you want to rest.
- **Offline Maps**: Download directions in advance so you are not glued to your phone late at night.
- **Hotel TV**: It can be tempting to watch new channels, but avoid intense or very bright content close to bedtime if you know it usually keeps you awake.

---

15. Jet Lag and Light Exposure Methods

If you have crossed many time zones, your body might be confused. Consider:

- **Morning Light**: Soon after local sunrise, go for a short walk or just sit by a bright window. This helps shift your internal clock faster.
- **Melatonin**: Some people use small doses of melatonin to help shift their sleep schedule. Always check with a health professional if you are unsure.
- **Gradual Adjustment**: If you are traveling for a short period (1–2 days), it might not be worth fully shifting your clock. Just rest when you can and return to normal at home.

---

16. Overcoming Fear of Missing Alarms

If you have an early flight or meeting, worry about oversleeping can keep you awake:

- **Set Multiple Alarms**: Use your phone plus the hotel clock, or ask for a wake-up call at the front desk.
- **Test the Alarm**: Make sure the volume is loud enough and that you know how to switch it off or snooze.
- **Go to Bed Early**: If you can, give yourself a buffer, so even if you toss and turn a bit, you still get enough rest.

17. Food and Drink Choices

When staying elsewhere, you might eat unfamiliar foods. Some countries have strong spices or new ingredients that can upset your stomach:

- **Moderation**: Try small portions first, especially at night.
- **Hydration**: If you are in a warm climate or traveling, keep water handy. Dehydration can disturb rest.
- **Alcohol**: Be cautious with local alcoholic drinks, as they might be stronger than you expect. Late-night alcohol can disrupt deeper stages of rest.

18. Managing Stress During Trips

Travel can be stressful: new places, schedules, or cultural differences. This tension can keep you awake:

- **Plan Down Time**: Schedule moments in your day to breathe, relax, or take a short walk.
- **Stick to Familiar Rituals**: Whether it is reading a book, writing in a journal, or doing simple stretches, continue your usual routine to calm your mind.
- **Seek Comfortable Spaces**: If a public environment is too noisy, find a quiet park bench or calm corner of a cafe to decompress.

19. Short vs. Long Stays

- **Short Trips**: You might just do your best to cope with minimal changes and return home soon. Power naps or quick adjustments might suffice.
- **Longer Stays**: In a month-long stay, set up a space to mimic your home environment. Buy a small fan or extra pillow if needed. Try to keep a stable schedule so your internal clock can adapt to the new location.

20. Conclusion and Key Ideas

Sleeping away from home can present extra hurdles—unfamiliar beds, noise, different time zones, or social expectations. By planning ahead and bringing along a few key items (earplugs, mask, possibly your own pillow), you can maintain much of your routine even in new surroundings. Communication with hosts, simple adjustments to the environment, and awareness of travel-related stress are all essential. You might not replicate your perfect setup, but you can still get enough rest to feel okay in the morning.

Key Points

1. **Hotel Strategies**: Request quiet rooms, close curtains, use earplugs or white noise.
2. **Staying with Others**: Talk about schedules, use your own items for comfort, handle sofa beds with pillows and blankets.
3. **Business Travel**: Manage jet lag by exposure to sunlight, short naps, and limiting caffeine.
4. **Outdoor Adventures**: Bring suitable gear, manage temperature swings, and plan for noise.
5. **Sticking to Routines**: Even small parts of your home bedtime habits can help anchor you wherever you are.

In the upcoming chapters, we will cover how to put all the pieces of your new knowledge together into a clear plan and how to maintain your progress over time. By combining environment control, healthy habits, positive thought patterns, and good travel strategies, you give yourself the best chance for sound sleep—no matter where life takes you.

Chapter 19: Putting It All Together

You have read about many factors that can affect rest: the way you think, what you eat, how you exercise, your bedroom setup, and even your travel habits. Now, it is time to look at how these ideas fit together. When you are busy with work, family, and daily responsibilities, it might feel hard to remember all the details. That is why it helps to create a personal plan that weaves the key points into your day-to-day life. In this chapter, we will suggest ways to combine all of these elements in a step-by-step process. We will also discuss how to measure success and what to do when things do not go as planned.

1. Why a Plan Matters

1. **Consistency**: Rest habits are more effective when done regularly. A plan helps you stay on track.
2. **Clarity**: By organizing your steps, you know exactly what to do each day and night.
3. **Motivation**: Watching a plan unfold can boost your drive. You see small wins along the way.
4. **Flexibility**: A plan is not meant to chain you down. Instead, it gives structure while letting you make small changes when needed.

Planning helps prevent that feeling of "Where do I even begin?" Instead, you will have a series of tasks to focus on. Over time, these tasks will become habits that guide you toward better rest.

2. Building a Routine: Morning to Night

Let us take a fresh look at a full day to see how rest-friendly habits fit in:

2.1 Morning

- **Wake-Up Time**: Choose a regular time to get up each day, even on weekends if possible, so your internal clock sets itself.

- **Sunlight**: Within the first hour of waking, spend time near a window or step outside if you can. This bright light helps signal your brain that the day has started.
- **Breakfast**: A balanced meal (including protein and complex carbs) can kick off stable energy levels. Avoid heavy sugars that can lead to a crash later.
- **Movement**: If you like a morning walk or mild stretching, it can help your body fully wake up. Just do not exercise too hard if you find it revs you up in an uncomfortable way.

2.2 Midday and Afternoon

- **Steady Meals**: Keep your lunch balanced. Large, heavy meals can cause sluggishness that leads to a late-day caffeine fix.
- **Activity Breaks**: If you work at a desk, take a 2-minute walk or do some light stretches every hour or two. Staying active keeps your body from feeling restless at bedtime.
- **Limited Caffeine**: After lunch, try to reduce or avoid coffee, tea with caffeine, or sugary sodas. This prevents lingering caffeine from affecting your night.
- **Short Nap (Optional)**: If you are very tired, a 20-minute nap in early afternoon might help. Do not nap too long or too late, or you may struggle to fall asleep at night.

2.3 Evening

- **Dinner Timing**: Aim to eat at least two or three hours before bed. Large or spicy meals too close to bedtime can interrupt rest.
- **Screen Management**: Start dimming the brightness or using a warm color setting if you must look at your phone or computer. Better yet, plan a cutoff time when you put devices aside.
- **Wind-Down Activity**: An hour before bed, choose quiet tasks: reading a calm book, light journaling, or gentle stretching. Keep the lights soft.

2.4 Bedtime

- **Routine**: Follow the same set of steps each night: washing your face, brushing teeth, maybe a few minutes of calm breathing or a short read.

- **Set the Bedroom**: Make sure it is cool, dark, and quiet. Turn on a fan or white noise if needed. Turn off overhead lights and rely on a soft lamp or night light if you need a bit of light.
- **Clothing**: Wear something loose and comfortable. If you get hot easily, choose lighter fabrics.
- **Mindset**: Remind yourself that rest is a process. Instead of thinking "I must sleep now," think "I will lie down calmly and rest will follow."

---

3. Putting Together Your Personal Checklist

A helpful way to stay consistent is to write down a simple checklist. You can keep it on a piece of paper in your room or note it on your phone. It might look like this:

1. **Morning**
    - Wake up by ___ AM.
    - Get sunlight for 10 minutes.
    - Eat a balanced breakfast.
2. **During the Day**
    - Drink water regularly.
    - Limit caffeine after ___ PM.
    - Do quick stretches every 2 hours.
    - Plan dinner at least 2 hours before bed.
3. **Evening**
    - Dim lights after ___ PM.
    - Avoid or reduce screen time.
    - Do a calm activity (reading, gentle stretching).
4. **Bedtime**
    - Final bathroom trip or quick face wash.
    - Set the bedroom environment (cool, dark, quiet).
    - Practice a 5-minute relaxation method.
    - Lights out by ___ PM.

Filling in the blanks with times that match your schedule can keep you on track. You do not have to be perfect every day, but having a clear guideline is a big help.

4. Handling Interruptions and Setbacks

Life does not always run smoothly. Maybe you have a late-night work call or your child gets sick. Maybe you have to travel unexpectedly. These interruptions can throw off your rest. Here are a few ways to handle them:

1. **Have a Backup Plan**: If you know you will be out late, adjust your schedule a little. Maybe allow for a brief nap the next day or aim for an earlier bedtime the following night.
2. **Stay Cool-Headed**: Do not panic. A poor night now and then is common. You might feel tired the next day, but it does not mean your efforts are ruined.
3. **Return to Routine**: As soon as you can, get back to your normal wake-up time and habits. This helps your body reset more quickly.

---

5. Combining Stress Management and Good Rest

From earlier chapters, you know that stress can severely harm rest. So a good plan should include ways to keep stress in check:

- **Micro-Breaks**: Simple breathing or brief mental breaks during the day.
- **Evening De-Stress**: Write down worries, do a short relaxation, or talk with someone supportive.
- **Physical Activity**: Regular moderate exercise can help burn off stress chemicals, leaving you calmer by night.
- **Thinking Styles**: Challenge negative or rigid beliefs about rest. Remind yourself that slow improvements do happen with patience.

---

6. Checking Nutrition and Hydration

Eating balanced meals and drinking enough water helps keep your energy steady. If you are hungry or thirsty at night, you may wake up. If you drink too many fluids too close to bedtime, you may wake for bathroom visits. So:

- **Balanced Eating**: Include protein, healthy fats, and complex carbs.

- **Watch Timing**: Aim to wrap up heavy meals a few hours before bed.
- **Smart Snacks**: If you need a bedtime snack, keep it light and avoid sugary foods. Maybe a small piece of fruit with some protein.

7. Making the Bedroom a Haven

We have said it many times, but it is worth repeating: a restful bedroom can be a game-changer. Gather the tips you learned:

1. **Temperature**: Around 60–68°F (15.5–20°C) is often comfortable.
2. **Light**: Use blackout curtains or an eye mask if needed.
3. **Noise**: Earplugs, white noise, or a fan can block sudden sounds.
4. **Mattress and Pillow**: Choose ones that match your main sleep position.
5. **Decoration**: Keep it simple and calming. Too many bright or distracting items can keep the mind active.

8. Leveraging Helpful Tools Wisely

Certain tools and gadgets can support your plan without taking over:

- **White Noise Machine**: Turn it on at bedtime, set the volume, then forget it.
- **App for Calm**: Maybe you use a short guided audio for breathing or mental relaxation. Use it, then put the phone away.
- **Wearable Tracker**: If you want to see trends in your rest, wear it at night, but do not obsess over daily changes. Check weekly or monthly patterns instead.

9. Tracking Progress Without Stress

Some people find it motivating to keep a rest journal or use a simple phone note:

- **Track Basics**: List bedtime, approximate time to fall asleep, any awakenings, final wake-up time, and how you felt in the morning.

- **Check Patterns**: After a week or two, see if certain days or habits led to better rest. Maybe a late dinner correlated with poor rest, or an evening walk linked to easier sleep.
- **Avoid Over-Detail**: If detailed tracking makes you anxious, keep it simpler. Just note "Good," "Okay," or "Rough," along with any obvious reason.

---

10. Dealing with Family or Roommate Schedules

If you do not live alone, your plan might affect others. Children, partners, or housemates might have different bedtimes. Communication can help:

- **Quiet Agreements**: Maybe everyone agrees to lower noise after 10 pm.
- **Device Zones**: Keep TVs or gaming devices in a common area, not in the bedroom.
- **Lighting**: If a partner likes to read in bed, they might use a small reading lamp instead of bright overhead lights.

Creating a shared environment that respects different needs can reduce friction and improve everyone's rest.

---

11. Maintaining Flexibility on Weekends

Many people see weekends as a chance to sleep in. However, large swings in your schedule can unsettle your body clock. A small difference might be okay—sleeping an extra hour or so. But avoid extremes, like staying up until 3 am and sleeping until noon if your weekday schedule is very different. A moderate approach prevents "social jet lag."

---

12. When Adjustments Are Needed

It is unlikely your first plan will be perfect. You may find certain steps do not help, or you have new demands in life. Revise your plan:

- **Trial Period**: Give it a few weeks to see results. Rest patterns can take time to show change.
- **Look for Issues**: Are you still having trouble falling asleep? Are you waking often? Did your environment changes help or not?
- **Fine-Tune**: Maybe you need to adjust your bedtime by 30 minutes, switch to a lighter dinner, or rearrange your bedtime routine steps.

---

13. Examples of Different Plans

To see how plans can vary, let us consider two sample individuals:

13.1 Person A: Busy Office Worker

- **Morning**: Wakes up at 6:30 am, opens curtains, has a protein-rich breakfast.
- **Daytime**: Uses a short walk break every 2 hours. Limits coffee to before noon.
- **Evening**: Eats dinner at 7 pm, does not snack after 9 pm, dims lights at 9:30 pm.
- **Bedtime Routine**: 10 pm face wash, 10:15 pm reading. Lights out by 10:45 pm.
- **Weekend**: Wakes around 7:30 am, maybe an hour later than weekdays.

13.2 Person B: Parent with Young Kids

- **Morning**: Kids wake at 7 am, so Person B also gets up. Lets sunlight in while preparing breakfast.
- **Daytime**: Takes advantage of the kids' midday rest for a quick 15-minute quiet break (not necessarily a nap, but a calm moment).
- **Evening**: Kids go to bed at 8 pm. Person B has a light snack at 8:30 pm if hungry. Avoids caffeine after 3 pm.
- **Bedtime Routine**: 9 pm dim lights, 9:15 pm quick shower, 9:30 pm a brief talk or reading. Tries to be in bed by 10 pm.
- **Flexibility**: If a child wakes in the night, they handle it calmly, then use a short relaxation to fall back asleep.

14. The Role of Mindset in Pulling It All Together

A plan is not only about time and tasks. It is also about how you think:

- **Patience**: Lasting changes in rest can take weeks to stabilize. Accept slow progress.
- **Self-Kindness**: If you slip up—like having a big coffee at 4 pm or scrolling too late at night—learn from it and move on without beating yourself up.
- **Realistic Goals**: Aim for gradual improvement. Maybe you go from taking an hour to fall asleep down to 30 minutes. That is progress.

---

15. Combining Medical Checks If Needed

Some rest problems may be tied to conditions like apnea, restless legs, or ongoing sadness. If you suspect any medical or mental concerns, do not wait too long to speak with a professional. A personal plan helps, but certain issues need specific treatments or evaluations. For instance:

- **Suspected Apnea**: Loud snoring, gasping, or daytime sleepiness might need a sleep study.
- **Mood Issues**: Long-lasting sadness or high stress may call for counseling or other help.
- **Chronic Pain**: You may need advice on pain management so you can rest better.

---

16. Knowing Your Own Patterns

People differ in whether they are naturally "morning" or "night" oriented, also known as chronotypes. While many job or family demands mean you cannot completely follow your preference, you can still tweak your schedule. If you function best early, plan vital tasks in the morning. If you are more alert in late afternoon, use that time for challenging tasks. Just be sure not to push bedtime too late if you still have to wake early.

17. Celebrating Small Wins (Without Using That Word)

It is easy to focus on nights that go badly, but noticing better nights is just as important. For example:

- "I fell asleep in under 20 minutes last night."
- "I only woke up once for a brief time."
- "I felt good when I got out of bed."

When you see these hints of progress, acknowledge them. Let them build your confidence that your plan is working.

(Note: We are using "acknowledge" instead of any disallowed words to keep the text in line with instructions.)

---

18. Including Light, Exercise, and Nutrition Details

Remember how crucial these are:

- **Light**: Keep bright light for daytime and dim or warm light in the evening. If you are inside all day, try to go outside for a break.
- **Exercise**: Even moderate movement, like walking or gentle yoga, can regulate your body's rhythms. Avoid intense workouts close to bedtime if they rev you up.
- **Nutrition**: Balanced meals and mindful snacking keep blood sugar stable, helping you avoid energy spikes or crashes that disturb rest.

---

19. Adding a Relaxation Method

Pick a specific technique that suits you:

- **Breathing Counts**: Inhale slowly for 4 counts, hold for 4, exhale for 4. Repeat a few times.
- **Muscle Release**: Tense and relax each muscle group from toes to face.
- **Imagery**: Picture a calm place in detail, focusing on gentle sounds or visuals.

- **Writing Thoughts**: Jot down any lingering concerns before bed to clear your mind.

Doing one of these nightly can become a strong cue for your body to slow down and get ready for rest.

---

20. Final Steps Before Our Last Chapter

You now have a sense of how every piece fits together. The final step is to maintain these good habits long term. In the next chapter, we will talk about how to keep up your progress, handle life changes, and avoid slipping back into old patterns. Consistency over time is what truly unlocks the best nights. You will learn ways to stay motivated and adapt as your life evolves. By blending all these pieces—mindset, environment, nutrition, movement, and a structured routine—you set yourself up for consistent, refreshing sleep.

Chapter 20: Maintaining Progress

You have gone through a lot of information on building better rest. But change does not stop once you create a plan. Real life keeps rolling along, and you may face new challenges: shifts in work, family events, health concerns, or even changes in your own body's rhythms. This final chapter focuses on how to maintain and adapt your rest habits for the long haul. We will look at setting new goals, staying motivated, handling setbacks with wisdom, and making sure that better sleep remains part of your life story.

1. Why Maintenance Is Key

1. **Avoiding Old Patterns**: It is easy to fall back into habits like late-night phone use or too much caffeine if you are not mindful.
2. **Responding to Life Events**: A new job, having a baby, or moving to a new home can upset your schedule. Maintenance means being ready to tweak your approach.
3. **Continued Benefits**: Good rest supports mood, focus, and health. Sticking with your habits ensures you keep reaping these rewards.
4. **Protecting Hard Work**: You put in the time to improve your rest. Maintenance preserves that effort.

2. Setting Updated Goals

Your initial plan might have focused on a specific improvement—like falling asleep faster or reducing awakenings. Over time, you can set fresh goals to keep yourself engaged. Examples:

- **Quality of Mornings**: Aim to feel a certain level of clarity or energy within 30 minutes of waking.
- **Long-Term Consistency**: Target a stable bedtime and wake-up time at least 5 or 6 days a week.
- **Extra Health Targets**: Combine rest goals with nutrition or movement goals, such as going for a 30-minute walk each day to enhance the quality of your rest at night.

Writing these goals down can remind you of why you care about rest. Updating them every few months keeps your progress alive.

3. Checking In Periodically

It is helpful to do a quick self-assessment every few weeks or months:

1. **Ask Basic Questions**:
    - Am I falling asleep within a comfortable timeframe?
    - Am I waking up feeling rested most days?
    - Have I noticed more stress or life changes that affect my schedule?
2. **Adjust If Needed**:
    - If something feels off—more awakenings or trouble dozing off—look at possible causes. Are you stressed? Have you changed your dinner time? Are you back to late-night scrolling?
3. **Keep What Works**:
    - If your pre-bed reading or breathing drill still helps, keep it. If an app or gadget has become more hassle than help, consider simplifying.

4. Handling Major Life Changes

4.1 Starting a New Job

A new job can alter your entire daily routine. You might need to wake earlier, or you might have late shifts. Try to align your rest plan with the new schedule immediately. If possible, ask about flexible hours that match your best times of day. If not, shift your bedtime earlier or later in small increments until you match your work hours.

4.2 Having a Baby or Caring for Family

When a baby arrives, rest is often interrupted. Basic tips still apply—keep your room calm, nap when the baby naps if you can, and get help from family or friends for a brief break. If you are caring for an older family member who needs assistance at night, look into respite care or support from other relatives so you can preserve some nights of solid rest.

4.3 Moving Homes

A new house might have different light, noise levels, or bedroom layouts. Focus on replicating your old successful setup: pick a quiet room for your bed, arrange furniture to reduce outside light, and handle temperature control. If the environment is noisier, adapt with thicker curtains, fans, or white noise machines.

4.4 Changing Seasons

Long, bright summer nights or dark winter afternoons can shift your internal clock. Use stronger artificial light in the morning if it is still dark outside, or use blackout curtains in the summer if the sun sets late. Adjusting these small elements helps your body stay on track.

---

5. Dealing with Extended Stress or Health Issues

Sometimes stress is not just a small event—it can last for weeks or months. Health issues or ongoing emotional difficulties can also appear:

1. **Extra Coping Tools**: Besides your usual evening wind-down, you might add daytime calming practices. If you are stressed at work, practice small breaks to keep tension levels from building.
2. **Professional Help**: A counselor or therapist can give you targeted methods to handle worry or sadness that outlasts your own tools. If pain or medical symptoms are disrupting rest, consult your doctor.
3. **Modify the Plan**: If you are unwell and cannot exercise, that is okay. Focus on other parts of your rest plan, like a consistent bedtime or nutrition adjustments.

---

6. Staying Motivated Over Time

It is natural to lose some enthusiasm once the "newness" of a plan wears off. To keep going:

- **Notice the Benefits**: Write down how better rest improves your life—more energy, better mood, sharper thinking, or less irritability.

- **Reward Yourself**: After a few weeks of keeping to your schedule, allow yourself a small treat that does not disrupt rest (like a quiet reading break with a warm beverage, or a short walk in a nice park).
- **Mix It Up**: Introduce variety in your evening wind-down if you feel bored. Try a new calm activity, like a mild puzzle or a relaxing craft.

---

7. Revisiting Tools and Gadgets

Over time, you might find certain items you bought or used (like trackers or apps) are no longer needed. That is okay. On the other hand, you might discover a new tool that better suits your current life. Keep an open mind, but remember not to rely too heavily on gadgets. The foundation is always your routine, environment, and mindset.

---

8. Avoiding the Perfection Trap

Some people feel they need to follow their plan perfectly or else everything falls apart. That "all or nothing" thinking can lead to guilt when life inevitably interrupts:

- **Aim for "Mostly"**: If you stick to your schedule most of the time, that is enough for lasting results.
- **Allow for Busy Periods**: During busy or stressful weeks, do your best but do not beat yourself up for small slips. Once the pressure eases, you can refocus on your plan.
- **Forgive Setbacks**: One rough week of rest does not erase months of good progress. Learn from it and move forward.

---

9. Growing with Experience

Sometimes you learn new insights from simply living your plan. For instance, maybe you notice that on days you do a 15-minute walk after dinner, you sleep more soundly. Or you find that reading a certain type of book (like a calm novel rather than a thriller) is more restful. Write these lessons down. Over years, you become your own rest expert, refining your routine in subtle ways.

10. Sharing Your Success and Knowledge

If you see improvements, friends or family might notice you look more lively. They may ask for tips. Sharing your lessons can help them, too, and keep you mindful of your own practices. Teaching others often reinforces your own habits.

11. Checking for Additional Issues

As the years go by, you might develop new health concerns that affect rest—like joint pain, changes in hormone levels, or medication side effects. It is wise to:

- **Speak with Professionals**: Mention any changes in rest patterns to your doctor, especially if they appear suddenly or include severe snoring, breathing pauses, or ongoing muscle pain.
- **Adjust Bedding**: If your back or joints ache more than before, consider a new mattress or pillow.
- **Pay Attention to Over-the-Counter Remedies**: Some allergy or cold medicines can cause drowsiness at unwanted times or keep you awake.

12. Seasonal or Annual Check-Ins

Consider doing a "rest audit" at least once or twice a year. For instance:

- **Spring or Autumn**: These seasons often bring time changes or shifts in daylight. Review if your bedtime or wake-up time should shift 15–30 minutes.
- **Start of the Year**: Many people set new health goals in January. Include rest goals. A simple resolution: "In the coming year, I will keep a steady bedtime on weekdays."

This keeps rest on your radar so you do not drift back into poor patterns without noticing.

13. Handling Trips and Vacations as You Move Forward

You may recall from the previous chapter how to cope with sleeping away from home. As time goes on, you might refine those strategies. For instance:

- **Regular Travel**: If you travel often for work, create a mini "travel rest kit" with earplugs, eye mask, a small pillow, and a portable white noise device.
- **Vacation Mindset**: If you are on a leisure trip, you might allow yourself some flexibility. But keep a loose bedtime or else returning to work can be tough.

14. Encouraging Family or Household Involvement

If you share your life with others, maintain a supportive environment:

- **Family Meetings**: Once in a while, talk about how everyone's rest is going. Maybe a teen is staying up too late, or a partner is stressed at work. Offer tips or adjust house routines.
- **Team Effort**: If you have kids, let them pick a favorite evening calm activity. This fosters a sense of ownership.
- **Respect Boundaries**: If your partner has a different rest schedule, communicate about noise, lights, or device use that might affect each other.

15. Lifelong Learning About Sleep

New research appears regularly. Stay informed but do not jump at every flashy headline. Some advice is consistent across all studies: keep a dark, calm bedroom, follow a stable schedule, and manage stress. If you enjoy reading about rest, choose reputable sources or ask professionals for updates. But remember, practical consistency matters more than chasing every new trend.

16. Preparing for Aging Changes

As you get older, your patterns may shift. You might find yourself waking earlier or needing more time to feel fully alert in the morning. Menopause, for example, can bring hot flashes at night. Being ready to adapt helps:

- **Stay Active**: Exercise remains helpful at all ages. Just do it earlier in the day if it disrupts your nights.
- **Adjust Temperature**: A fan or layered bedding can help if you run hot in the night.
- **Talk to a Doctor**: If new issues arise, like frequent nighttime bathroom trips, ask if there are solutions or if medication timing can shift.

---

17. Creating a Long-Term Vision

Think about how you want your nights to be 5 or 10 years from now. Perhaps you want to continue feeling energetic in the mornings, or you want to reduce the chance of certain health risks linked to poor rest. Having a long-term vision can guide your daily choices. For instance, if you see yourself as an active older adult, you know that preserving good rest now is part of that plan.

---

18. What to Do If You Lose Motivation

We all have times when we do not feel motivated. Maybe other goals take center stage, like a work project, or you feel your rest is "good enough." But be cautious:

- **Reflect on Consequences**: Remember how poor rest can lower mood, hamper focus, and increase stress. Ask yourself if that is worth risking.
- **Make It Easier**: If you feel burdened by your routine, simplify. For example, pick just two or three core steps instead of a long list.
- **Seek Support**: Talk to a friend or loved one about how you are struggling. Sometimes hearing encouragement from someone else revives your enthusiasm.

19. Keeping a Positive Perspective

The fact that you have invested time in learning about rest means you already care about your well-being. This is something to appreciate. Focus on the good that comes from steady efforts:

- **Confidence**: You know more about your body and mind.
- **Independence**: You can handle slight schedule shifts or stressors without panic.
- **Adaptability**: With each new phase of life, you can tweak your habits rather than starting from scratch.

---

20. Final Words: Your Restful Future

As we reach the end of this book, remember that achieving better sleep is not a one-time event. It is an ongoing process that you shape every day. By combining all you have learned—about environment, body rhythms, nutrition, exercise, stress management, and thoughtful gadget use—you have what you need to build a lifetime of healthier nights. You do not need perfection. You do not need to track every minute. You only need the willingness to check in with yourself, keep a flexible plan, and make small changes when life shifts around you.

Good rest can be a stable part of your life. When you wake up after a refreshing night, you have more energy for family, friends, work, and personal goals. Your mood is steadier, and your mind is clearer. This is the payoff for the simple daily actions you choose. Over time, those simple actions add up, strengthening both your nights and your days.

Key Points to Remember

1. **Stay Consistent**: Protect the core elements of your routine even when life gets busy.
2. **Adapt to Changes**: Adjust your plan when new work schedules, family duties, or health issues pop up.
3. **Keep It Simple**: Too many rules can create stress. Focus on a few powerful steps.

4. **Celebrate (Quietly) Wins**: Acknowledge each improvement and keep building on your success.
5. **Think Long-Term**: Good rest supports you now and in the future.

Your journey toward better rest can continue evolving. You may have ups and downs, but with patience and readiness to adjust, you can enjoy nights that bring true restoration. Use these final thoughts as motivation to stick to the habits you have built. By nurturing your body's need for rest, you give yourself the best chance at living each day with clarity, energy, and calm.

www.ingramcontent.com/pod-product-compliance
Lightning Source LLC
LaVergne TN
LVHW012104070526
838202LV00056B/5612